Atlas of Otoscopy

Atlas of Otoscopy

JACK L. PULEC, MD
Clinical Professor of Otolaryngology, Head and Neck Surgery
University of Southern California
School of Medicine
Clinical Professor of Otolaryngology, Head and Neck Surgery
Loma Linda University
Editor-in-Chief
The *Ear, Nose and Throat Journal*
President
Ear International
President, Pulec Ear Clinic
Los Angeles, California

CHRISTIAN DEGUINE, MD
Retired, Otolaryngologist
Gap, France

SINGULAR
THOMSON LEARNING ™

Australia Canada Mexico Singapore Spain United Kingdom United States

MW

SINGULAR

THOMSON LEARNING

Atlas of Otoscopy
by Jack L. Pulec, MD, and Christian Deguine, MD

Business Unit Director:
William Brottmiller

Acquisitions Editor:
Marie Linvill

Editorial Assistant:
Kristin Banach

Executive Marketing Manager:
Dawn Gerrain

Channel Manager:
Tara Carter

Executive Production Manager:
Karen Leet

Production Editor:
Sandy Doyle

Library of Congress Cataloging-in-
Publication Data
Pulec, Jack L. (Jack Lee), 1932A
Atlas of Otoscopy/by Jack L. Pulec and
    Christian Deguine
p. ; cm.
Includes index.
ISBN 0-7693-0011-1 (hardcover; includes
    index)
1. Otoscopy—Atlases. 2. Ear—Diseases—
Atlases. I. Deguine, Christian. II. Title.
[DNLM: 1. Diagnostic Techniques,
Otological—Atlases.
WV 17 P981a 2001]
RF123.P85.2001
6718'07565—dc21 00-030127

NOTICE TO THE READER

11/21/02

Contents

Section IV: Acute Otitis Media   **37**

Section V: Disease of the Tympanic Membrane   **45**

Section VI: Serous Otitis Media   **55**

Foreword

A Chinese saying goes as follows: "It is better to see one time, than to listen one hundred times." This is a strange way to start an appreciation in a book of otology, but not really, as this book is a collection of photographs as a means of learning in the field of otology. For sure, a really good photograph shows more than a few sentences, and above all describes much better. This is all the more true when the master who has taken the pictures is named Christian Deguine.

Christian Deguine is not only the most sincere person I have ever met in my life but is also one of the most talented surgeons I know and by far the most important pioneer in the photography of ear pathology. He has helped to develop its technology and in Europe he is recognized for having developed for the first time an impressive collection of external and middle-ear slides, of all kinds of pathology. Every slide of his extensive collection is signed by his name in the lower right-hand corner as follows, "Col. Christian Deguine."

I remember, one day at an ear, nose, and throat meeting a young student, sitting beside me, who asked: "Is he a Colonel in the army?" I answered, "Col. stands for collection." But nobody in the world has made a collection of slides more impressive in both number and quality.

Jack Pulec is the ideal partner for such a book, not only because he is Editor-In-Chief of the *Ear, Nose and Throat Journal*, not only because they are good friends, but also because, if there is a clone of Christian Deguine in the United States of America, it is he.

So, my thoughts go again to the young student in the ear, nose, and throat field and to all who want to learn about external and middle-ear pathology. This book is a beautiful and extremely efficient way to learn.

I have a deep admiration for what Jack and Christian have achieved and feel privileged to have written a few lines about their masterful work.

Docteur Jean-Bernard Causse

Preface

Interpretation and understanding of what is seen through the otoscope requires significant training, study, and practice. Indeed, it is often more than 3 months of diligent work before a resident in otolaryngology begins to understand what is being seen other than a colorful mass at the end of a small tunnel. It is even more difficult for physicians in other disciplines to learn to interpret what is seen otoscopically. The unusual popularity and extreme success of The Otoscopic Clinics published monthly in the *Ear, Nose and Throat Journal* as well as the Rhinoscopic Clinics and Laryngoscopic Clinics have led us to produce three atlases made up of a compilation of these clinics published during the last 7½ years and, in addition, clinics that are yet to be published. The value of this atlas is that the otoscopic photographs are of the highest quality and have been taken and interpreted by successful senior otologists.

This atlas contains at least one example of almost every important abnormality or condition likely to be seen by an examining physician. The commentary that accompanies each photograph describes in detail exactly what can and cannot be seen. The implications of the pathology and the best treatment are briefly summarized.

This atlas should be useful to anyone who practices otoscopy. This includes not only otologists, otolaryngologists, and residents in otolaryngology training, but also pediatricians, general practitioners, internists, audiologists, and hearing aid dispensers. Practitioners who use a telescope for otoscopy and create a print can compare the print with photographs in this atlas to obtain the best understanding of the pathology and best treatment. All conditions encountered in a general practice are included that involve the external auditory canal, tympanic membrane, middle ear, and different types of mastoid cavities.

A special effort has been made to describe the different types of chronic suppurative otitis media and to clarify the specific treatment that offers the highest level of success with the least amount of surgery.

The overwhelming majority of photographs were supplied by the authors. A few valuable photographs published in the *Ear, Nose and Throat Journal* were provided by other physicians, who are identified in footnotes. We gratefully acknowledge their contributions.

We gratefully acknowledge the diligent secretarial help and proofreading of Marilyn L. Lewis. We thank Marlene B. Pulec who proofread the majority of the text.

We appreciate the help of Mr. John H. Whaley III and Mr. Mark Goodman of the *Ear, Nose and Throat Journal* for making the initial publication of these illustrations possible and for allowing the material to be published in this atlas. We also gratefully acknowledge Ms. Candice Janco, Sandy Doyle, and Dr. Sadanand S. Singh of Singular Publishing Group for the outstanding way that they have treated this material and made it available to our readers.

Jack L. Pulec, MD
Christian Deguine, MD

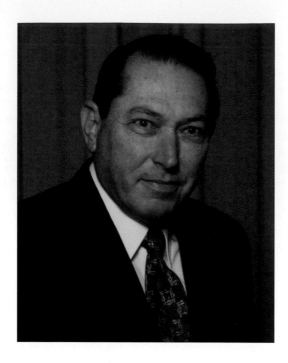

Jack L. Pulec, MD

Jack L. Pulec, MD, is Clinical Professor of Otolaryngology, Head and Neck Surgery at the University of Southern California School of Medicine in Los Angeles and at Loma Linda University School of Medicine. He is the Founder and President of Ear International and the Pulec Ear Clinic in Los Angeles, California where he confines his full-time practice to otology and neuro-otology. Dr. Pulec has been active in teaching advanced neuro-otologic surgery and diagnosis throughout the world. He travels extensively, lectures, and has performed surgery on six continents. He is on the editorial board of several scientific journals and has made a large number of scientific contributions, including original papers, book chapters, books, editorials, posters, movies, and videotapes. He is Editor-in-Chief of the *Ear Nose and Throat Journal*. Dr. Pulec has been listed in *The Best Doctors in America, Who's Who in America,* and the Town and Country Exclusive Directory "The Best Medical Specialists in the U.S." He has received many honors including the 1998 Practitioner of Excellence Award of the Board of Governors of the American Academy of Otolaryngology—Head and Neck Surgery.

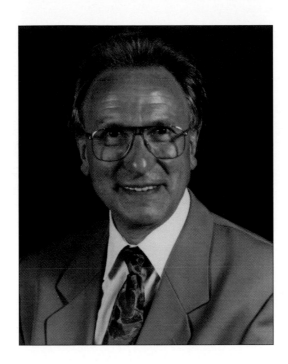

Christian DeGuine, MD

Christian Deguine, MD, is retired from the active practice of medicine and lives in Gap, France. He worked the major part of his career in Lille, France where he confined his practice to otology. The unique nature of his practice allowed him to concentrate on the treatment of chronic otitis media and to perform possibly more operations for this condition than any other surgeon. Throughout his practice, Dr. Deguine has been an enthusiastic teacher, worldwide lecturer, and has made many valuable contributions to the scientific literature, including co-authorship of the book *Les greffes du tympan* in 1990 and the CD *Pathologie de l'oreille moyenne* in 2000.

Dr. Deguine has long been interested in photography, composing a shot, adjusting the light, and doing his own developing and printing with the skill of a professional. The advent of the Hopkins' optical system used with a Karl Storz lens and light system made photography of the tympanic membrane practical. With two camera systems used every day, Dr. Deguine became the world's foremost otoscopic photographer.

Dedication

To my wife, Chantel, with love and thanks for her patience.

This book would not have seen the light of day without her silence during so many hours spent in the photolab.

Christian DeGuine, MD

Dedication

To Marlene, my wife, best friend, companion, and invaluable muse.

Jack L. Pulec, MD

SECTION I

Normal Ear

1

Normal Tympanic Membrane

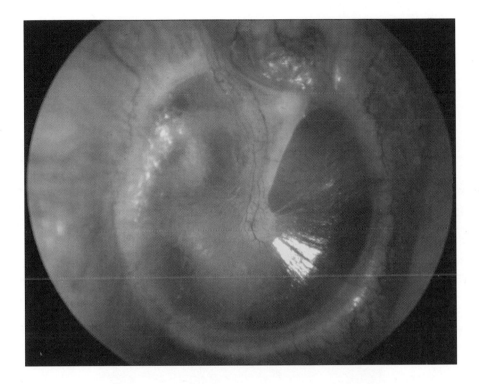

Fig 1–1

These otoscopic views depict completely normal tympanic membranes.[1,2] The external auditory canal is unobstructed and free from any lesion. The pars tensa is translucent and free from any perforation or healed perforation. There is no evidence of tympanosclerosis. The annular ring is intact. The pars tensa is intact and shows no evidence of retraction. The malleus is seen from the umbo at the direct center of the tympanic membrane along its long handle extending vertically in a superior direction to the short process, a whitish protrusion near the superior part of the tympanic membrane. Capillaries and blood vessels are seen as they begin near the malleus and extend in a radial fashion superiorly and especially posteriorly. The cream-colored spot representing the bone of the promontory on the medial wall of the tympanum is seen through the center of the membrane. The dark spot seen through the membrane anteriorly is the tubotympanum. A smaller and not so dark spot seen behind the posterior inferior quadrant represents the round window niche. A slightly pink cylindrical nerve, the chorda tympani, can be seen through the posterior superior quadrant of the membrane between the handle of the malleus and the annulus. The incus and stapes can also be seen inferior to the chorda tympani. A light reflex, a white patch, is seen reflecting from near the center of the pars tensa and the pars flaccida.

References

1. Deguine C. L'examen otoscopique. *NPN Med.* 1983;3: 781–789.
2. Deguine C. Otoscopic photography. In: *Recent Advances in Otolaryngology.* London: Churchill Livingstone; 1995:7:19–26.

2

Otoscopic Anatomy:
Items Visible on the Surface

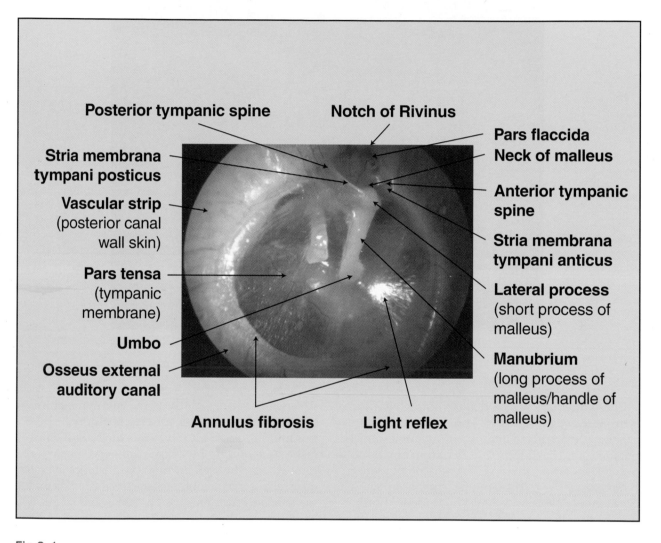

Fig 2–1

3

Otoscopic Anatomy: Structures Visible Through the Translucent Tympanic Membrane

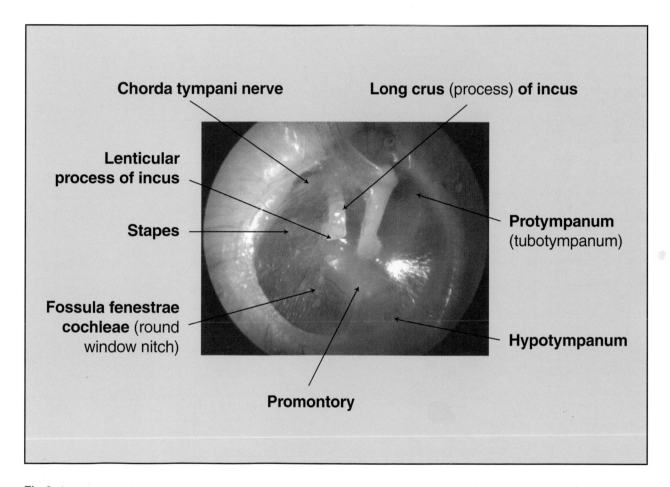

Fig 3–1

Bibliography

Bast TH, Anson BJ. *The Temporal Bone and the Ear*. Springfield, Ill: Charles C Thomas; 1949.

Proctor B. *Surgical Anatomy of the Ear and Temporal Bone*. New York, NY: Thieme Medical Publishers; 1989.

SECTION II

Abnormal Tympanic Membrane— Functionally Normal

4

Myringostapedopexy

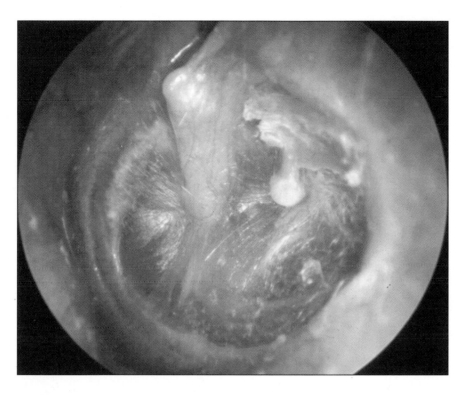

Fig 4–1

The otoscopic view is that of a left ear with a clearly abnormal appearance in an asymptomatic patient. Hearing is normal. This represents a myringostapedopexy. The short process of the malleus is the white structure at the top of the photograph. Extending vertically, inferiorly to the short process is the long process of the malleus. To the right of the umbo is a small white structure representing the lenticular process of the incus or capitulum of the stapes. The pars flaccida is adherent to this struc-ture, thereby conducting sound to the inner ear. The long process of the incus appears to be eroded. Superiorly, a small amount of epithelial debris can be seen. Myringostapedopexy, when it occurs natu-rally, can be stable and function well. When hearing is normal, no treatment is necessary. Creation of myringostapedopexy surgically on purpose has been very difficult to accomplish. Other methods of ossicular reconstruction have been found to be more successful.

5

Tympanosclerosis (Cosmetic)

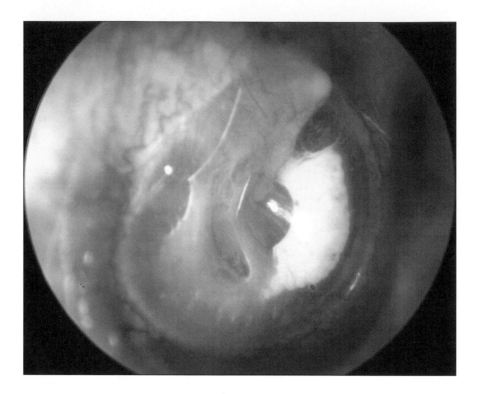

Fig 5–1

The otoscopic view is of a right ear demonstrating a solitary area of tympanosclerosis within the anterior half of the pars tensa. The white mass within the middle layer of the tympanic membrane causes no hearing loss. The posterior half of the tympanic membrane demonstrates a patchy, opaque appearance indicative of scar formation and healing from old infection. No treatment is required in the absence of hearing loss.

Bibliography

Pulec JL, Kinney SE. Diseases of the tympanic membrane. In: Paparella MM, Shumrick DA, eds. *Otolaryngology*. Vol 2. Philadelphia, Pa: W. B. Saunders Company; 1973:55–74.

6

Minimal Tympanosclerosis (Cosmetic)

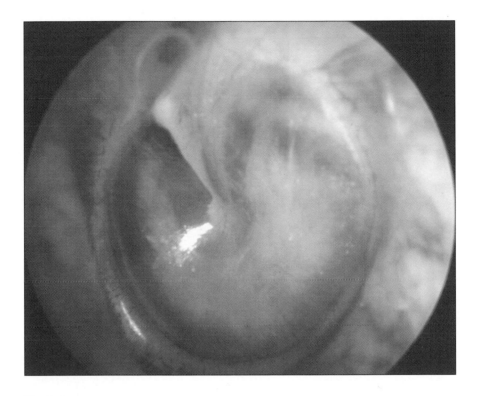

Fig 6–1

This otoscopic view is of the left ear in a patient with no symptoms or complaints. The only abnormality is a slight, patchy, opaque appearance of the pars tensa. The ear is well aerated and there is no infection. The chorda tympani and the incus can be seen through the pars tensa in the posterior, superior quadrant. In the absence of hearing loss or other complaint, this ear requires no treatment. It probably represents a very mild form of tympanosclerosis.

7

Patchy Tympanosclerosis (Cosmetic)

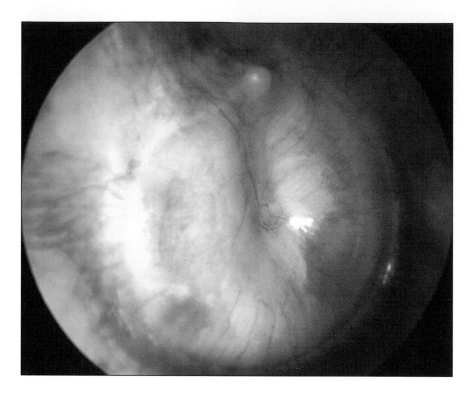

Fig 7–1

The otoscopic view is that of a right ear in a patient without symptoms or hearing loss. The pars tensa has patches of opaque, white-appearing material as well as a small area anteriorly of near-normal appearance. The tympanosclerosis here is cosmetic and requires no treatment or routine follow-up in the absence of complaint by the patient.

8

Asymptomatic Tympanosclerosis

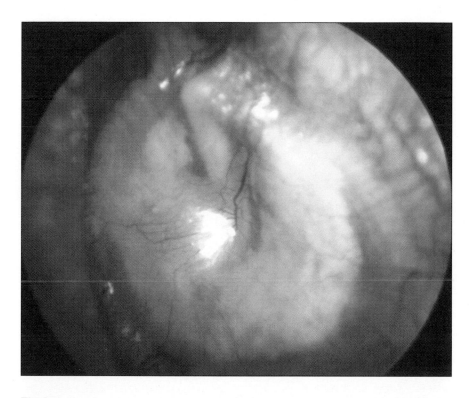

Fig 8–1

This is the otoscopic view of a left ear in a patient with no complaints or findings. The long process of the malleus is seen as it lies vertically in the superior half of the pars tensa. The entire pars tensa is moderately opaque, preventing structures within the tympanum from being seen. In the absence of an ossicular fixation or a tympanic membrane producing hearing loss, no treatment or routine follow-up is required. The tympanosclerosis is cosmetic and represents an abnormality but does not constitute pathology that requires treatment.

9

Healed Neomembrane and Tympanosclerosis

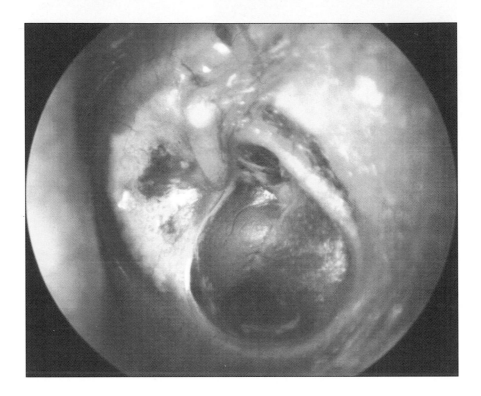

Fig 9–1

This is the otoscopic view of a left ear in a patient with no complaint. Hearing is normal despite the abnormal appearance of the tympanic membrane. A large, healed perforation with the two-layered membrane is seen in the posterior half of the pars tensa. At the upper edge of the perforation, the chorda tympani passes over the incus and stapes. Anterior to the vertical long process of the malleus is the pars tensa, which is involved with tympanosclerosis. Occasionally, this neomembrane may rupture during swimming or diving and tympanoplasty may be required. In the absence of symptoms, however, no treatment is required.

10

Tympanosclerosis (Cosmetic) and Retraction

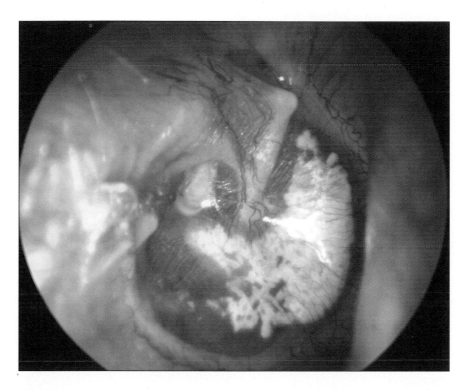

Fig 10–1

The otoscopic view is that of a right ear in an asymptomatic patient. A large area of tympanosclerosis involves the anterior and inferior portions of the pars tensa. This is cosmetic and is not producing fixation of the tympanic membrane or the ossicular chain. There is slight retraction over the incus. The pars flaccida anterior to the malleus is also slightly retracted. At the posterior annulus and external auditory canal an accumulation of cerumen is present. Although this ear should have regular, routine observation to detect any progression of the retraction of the pars tensa, it is probably stable and requires no treatment.

11

Dehiscence of Superior External Auditory Canal Wall Bone

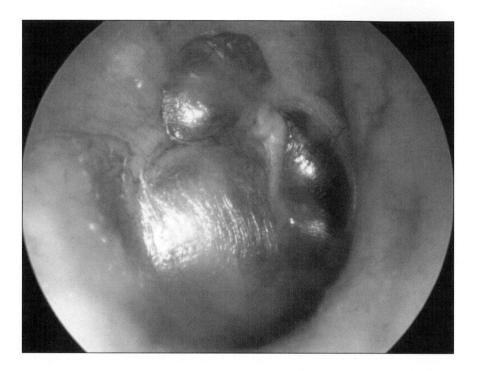

Fig 11–1

The otoscopic view is of a right ear which is functionally normal. The first impression is that the anatomy is normal. Closer observation reveals that the notch of Rivinus is significantly larger than normal. There is no retraction of the pars flaccida into the epitympanum. The head and neck of the malleus are visible through the pars flaccida. A 0.5-mm white spot of tympanosclerosis is anterior to the umbo. Three separate areas have a light reflex, one on the pars flaccida superior to the chorda tympani nerve, one on the anterior superior quadrant of the pars tensa, and the largest, brightest one on the posterior superior quadrant of the pars tensa. Both membranes are bulging outward because of middle-ear inflation shortly before this photograph was taken.

SECTION III

Diseases of the External Auditory Canal

12

Impacted Cerumen

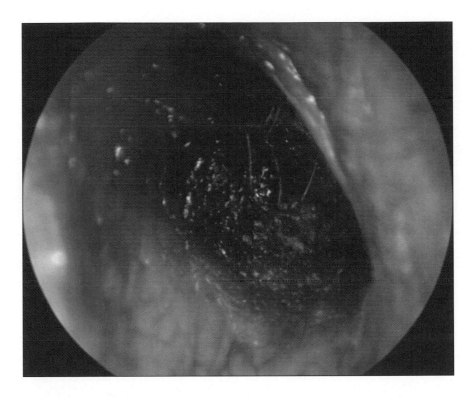

Fig 12–1

This is the otoscopic view of a right ear with a large, dark brown mass of hard cerumen completely occluding the external auditory canal. The mass is visible at the bony cartilaginous junction of the external auditory canal. The hard cerumen contains hairs, which act as a reinforcement of the cerumen. Impacted cerumen is a common cause of temporary hearing loss, tinnitus, and ear fullness. The etiology is unknown. Many methods are available to remove the impacted cerumen. The consistency of the cerumen determines which technique will work best. A hard mass as demonstrated in the photograph is usually best removed with a ring curette and use of the operating microscope. A softer, more liquid type of cerumen is usually best removed by irrigating the ear with water of body temperature. Difficult-to-remove cerumen may sometimes be softened by the installation into the ear of an edible oil or mineral oil for several days. In cases in which the impacted cerumen produces otalgia, the ear canal can first be anesthetized by injection of a local anesthetic followed by painless removal in a surgical manner using the operating microscope. A lytic agent such as Cerumenex may be used for several days to liquify difficult-to-remove cerumen.

13

Beach Sand in the Ear

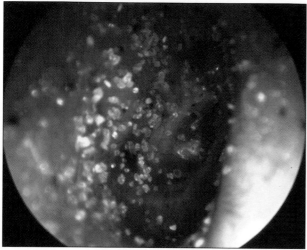

Fig 13–1. Right ear.

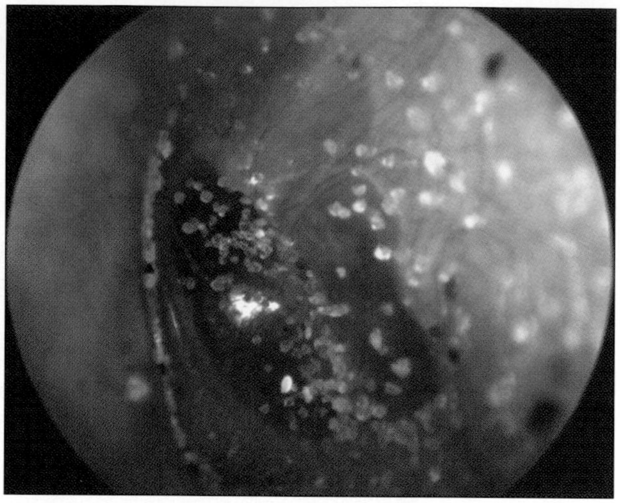

Fig 13–2. Left ear.

The otoscopic views are of completely normal ears of a patient who had been at the beach. Both external auditory canals and tympanic membranes are entirely normal with the exception of the white grains of sand. The self-cleaning mechanism of the ear will carry the sand to the meatus within a few weeks. Should the patient complain of hearing loss or ear fullness, the otologist can remove the sand with water lavage.

14

Foreign Body (Tooth) in the External Auditory Canal*

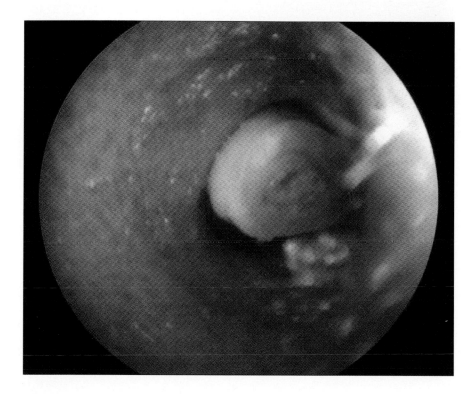

Fig 14–1

The otoscopic photograph shows a deciduous tooth in the external auditory canal. It is of a 4-year-old girl who excitedly woke up one morning and checked under her pillow to see what the tooth fairy had left her. She felt a rather strange sensation in her left ear, because her tooth had some how managed to lodge itself in the left external auditory canal. Following photography the tooth was removed without incident and the tooth fairy was able to accomplish her mission. Removal of a foreign body from an ear canal can be hazardous and it is best performed by a surgeon trained in microscopic ear surgery and with the correct instruments. In an uncooperative young child a general anesthetic may be required. For an adult, if removal is painful,

the canal can first be anesthetized by a local injection after which the foreign body can be removed in the office. It is not uncommon for children to place their teeth in their ear canals and usually the crown faces the tympanic membrane and the sharp concave end of the tooth where the fang or root has been eroded faces toward the exterior making the removal more difficult in the face of any canal skin edema. Removal of foreign bodies from the external auditory canal can be done by the skilled otologist using the proper equipment without injury to the tympanic membrane, ossicular chain, or inner ear.

*Photograph courtesy of Jack B. Anon, MD, Erie, Pennsylvania.

15

Furunculosis*

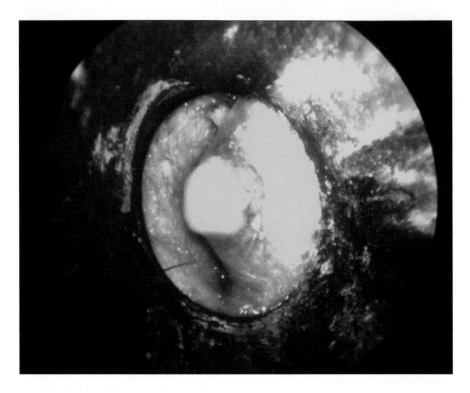

Fig 15–1

Furunculosis of the external auditory canal arises from a small localized infection involving a hair follicle. The condition occurs in the outer third of the ear canal where hair follicles are located. The patient with a furuncle usually has otalgia and fever. The affected region may be tender to touch, possibly with palpable, tender regional lymphadenitis. Otoscopy reveals a tender abscess. Furuncles are commonly found between the junction of the tragus and the anterior crus of the helix. Depending on the stage of the disease process, the abscess may be either superficial and pointed or deep and diffuse.[1] The unaffected eardrum may not be seen in cases in which the furuncle is large or when it is associated with a diffuse otitis externa. If the infection involves a group of follicles, the coalescent abscess becomes a large carbuncle.

Staphylococcus aureus is the usual causative organism.[2] Systemic antibiotics should be employed in the earlier stages, consisting of either a beta-lactamase-resistant penicillin or a quinolone derivative such as Ciprofloxacin. Definitive treatment consists of incision and drainage of the furuncle. The pus should be submitted for bacteriological culture and sensitivity. The follicular abscess may either be allowed to drain spontaneously, aided by frequent applications of a hot pad, or incised under local anesthesia if the abscess is fluctuant but not yet discharging.

Once the abscess is opened and the pus expressed, the condition rapidly resolves. Topical antibiotic ear drops covering the appropriate organism should be applied and the incised area kept clean. An otowick or antibiotic-impregnated wick may be inserted temporarily if there is significant ear canal edema and narrowing. Adequate analgesia should be made

*Chapter contributed by K. L. Chan, MMBS; G. Soo, FRCS (Glasgow), and C. A. van Hasselt, MMed(Otol) from the Division of Otorhinolaryngology, Department of Surgery, Prince of Wales Hospital, Shatin, Hong Kong.

available for this painful condition and nocturnal sedation may also be required.

If there is no response to conventional treatment, drug sensitivities should be reviewed. Multi-drug-resistant *S. aureus* infection, diabetes mellitus, or an underlying immune deficiency must be excluded as potential causes of persistent or recurrent infections.

References

1. Jahn AF, Hawke M. Infections of the external ear. In: Cummings CW, Fredrickson JM, Harker LA, et al, eds. *Otolaryngology—Head and Neck Surgery*. 2nd ed. St. Louis, Mo: Mosby Year Book; 1993:2790–2794.
2. Lucente FE, Lawson W. Novick NL. *The External Ear*. Philadelphia, Pa: W. B. Saunders Company; 1995.

16

Keratinized Epithelial Folds in the External Auditory Canal*

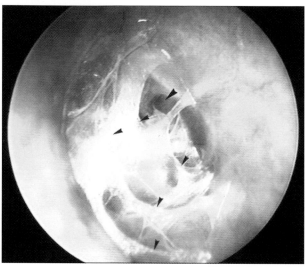

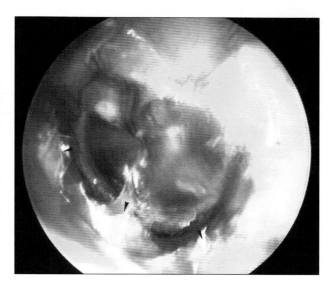

Fig 16–1. Multiple thin, keratinized epithelial folds arise circumferentially from the left eardrum and external auditory canal (small arrows). The pars flaccida, the handle of the malleus, and the long process of the incus (large arrow) can be seen.

Fig 16–2. The left eardrum and the residual keratinized epithelium (small arrows) in the external auditory canal after removal of the epithelial folds.

This endoscopic image of the left external auditory canal was taken from a 37-year-old Chinese woman who had complained of tinnitus in her left ear for 1 year. Other than the ringing sound, which was worse at night, she had no other ear symptoms such as hearing loss, otalgia, or otorrhea. She denied scratching her ears, using cotton swabs, or applying any topical medication to her left ear. No previous otologic surgery had been performed. She had seen many doctors, who had apparently diagnosed perforations, a retraction pocket of the eardrum, and chronic otitis media.

Eventually, she was seen by one of the authors.

On examination, her hearing was normal, as shown by a free-field voice test. Tuning fork tests were also normal. However, otoscopic examination of her left ear showed multiple thin, keratinized epithelial folds arising from the tympanic membrane and the external auditory canal.

*This chapter was contributed by Peter K. M. Ku, FRCS(Ed), John N. Marshall, FRCS(Eng) and Andrew van Hasselt, FCS(SA), MMed(Otol), Division of Oto-rhinolaryngology, Department of Surgery, The Chinese University of Hong Kong, Prince of Wales Hospital, Shatin, New Territories, Hong Kong.

17

Otomycosis With Pus

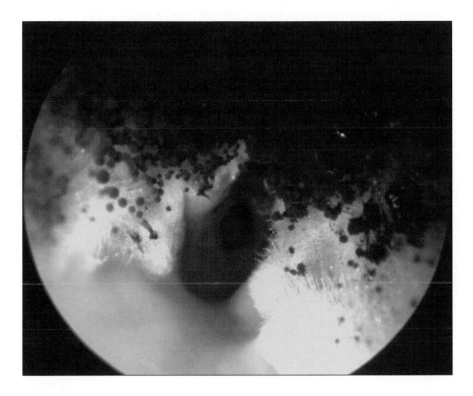

Fig 17–1

The otoscopic view is that of a right ear demonstrating a 20%, dry central perforation of the pars tensa and extensive acute otitis externa with frons of both white and black fungi. The floor or the external auditory canal is covered with thick, cream-colored pus. Otomycosis is a result of secondary invasion of the ear canal, and when a perforation is present, also the invasion of middle ear when conditions are right. Fungi are not the primary problem and are usually easily eradicated. Treatment is profuse and frequent irrigation of the involved ear with vinegar. Fungi cannot survive in an acid environment. Occasionally, antifungal ear drops or Cresylate ear drops can be useful. After the ear has become dry, surgical repair of the perforation and education of the patient in the proper toilette of the ear canal to keep it dry by the use of rubbing alcohol after swimming is usually successful in the prevention of recurrence.

18

Otomycosis

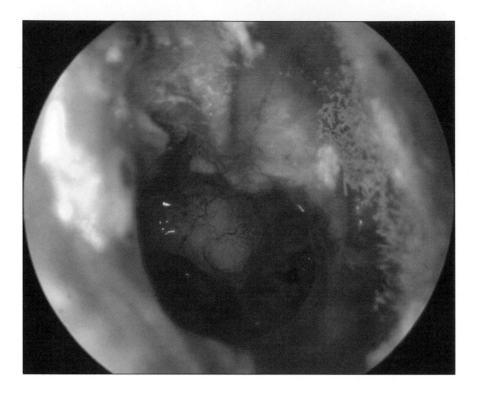

Fig 18–1

The otoscopic view shows a right ear with a 90% perforation of the pars tensa. The tympanum appears dry. The malleus extends from the superior annulus inferiorly and the capitulum of the stapes and lenticular process of the incus are seen at the left upper quadrant. A bluish-gray mass of mycelia and a white mass of mycelia are seen on the anterior canal wall. Dried yellow pus is on the posterior canal wall skin. Treatment involves profuse frequent irrigation of the ear with 4% acetic acid (plain, white household vinegar) and subsequent tympanoplasty to correct the perforation. Treatment of otomycosis is topical. Systemic antifungal agents are rarely, if ever, required or valuable.

19

Flourishing Otomycosis*

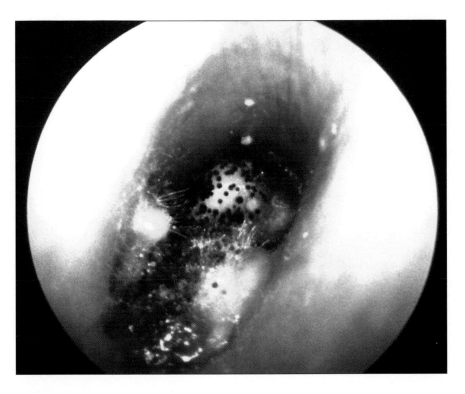

Fig 19–1

This endoscopic view shows the right ear of a patient with a history of chronic otitis externa to whom long-term topical antibiotic steroid ear drops had been administered. In addition to a deep-seated itchiness, he also complained of scant odorless discharge. The diagnosis of otomycosis caused by *Aspergillus niger* was made immediately after otoscopic examination.

Otomycosis accounts for about 9% of otitis externa, and is occasionally associated with bacterial infection.[1] Most cases result from *A. niger* infection, although other causative organisms, including *Candida* and *Penicillium*, have been reported. Cutaneous aspergillosis is more common in tropical and subtropical areas that experience long periods of high atmospheric humidity, such as Hong Kong, Nigeria, and Egypt.[2] Predisposing factors to fungal infection include habitual instrumentation, dermatitis, and immunocompromising conditions. Itching is the main manifestation of this condition,

followed by discomfort, tinnitus, hearing impairment, and discharge.[3]

Contrary to other fungi, *A. niger* is the only organism that can be correctly identified by the characteristic appearance of the ear canal. A whitish, fluffy, cottonlike material consisting of fungal hyphae and dusky black conidiophores, together with epithelial debris and exudate deep in the ear canal, is the hallmark of this condition. Confirmation by culture of the material in a moist potassium hydroxide (KOH) preparation is needed only in exceptional cases.

Treatment should include careful removal of the debris by microscopic aural toilette and application of topical antifungal agents with an acid pH. As the mycelia extend below the necrotic surface and invade the deeper layers of the tissue, to achieve adequate cleaning the debris should be completely removed, often resulting in contact bleeding. In cases of mixed bacterial and fungal infection, combined treatment with topical antibiotics and antifungal agents is required. Equally important, the patient should be advised to keep the ear dry and avoid overuse of therapeutic ear preparations.

References

1. Mugliston T, O'Donoghue. Otomycosis—a continuing problem. *J Laryngol Otol.* 1985;99:327–333.
2. Tang HMK. Acute otitis externa in Hong Kong—a prospective study. *Hong Kong Pract.* 1983;(February): 446–453.
3. Than KM, Naing KS, Min M. Otomycosis in Burma, and its treatment. *Am J Tropical Med Hyg.* 1980;29: 620–623.

*This chapter was contributed by Martin Wai Pak, FRCS (Edin), Gordon Soo, FRCS(Glasg), and Charles Andrew van Hasselt, MMED(Otol), FCS(SA) from the Division of Otorhinolaryngology, Department of Surgery, Prince of Wales Hospital, Shatin, Hong Kong.

20

Acute External Otitis

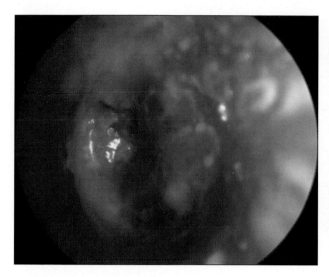

Fig 20–1

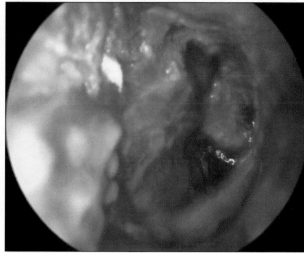

Fig 20–2

The otoscopic views are of the right and left ears of a 24-year-old woman with otorrhea, otalgia, and normal hearing following swimming. In this case, it also could be called "swimmer's ear." Acute external otitis is characterized by ear pain and otorrhea. Physical examination reveals a very tender ear with any manipulation of the pinna or external auditory canal. The otoscopic view of each ear reveals an intact tympanic membrane covered with debris. The external auditory canal skin, however, is edematous and macerated. In its worst stage, the external auditory canal can be completely occluded by edema of the skin and excoriation and edema can extend to the pinna and to tissues surrounding the

external auditory canal. Treatment usually involves local heat, analgesics, and topical administration of a water-soluble combination of antibiotics and steroids. In cases where the ear canal is occluded because of severe edema, a cotton wick is placed in the ear canal to allow the topical medication to reach the involved skin. The cotton is kept moist with the administration of two drops each hour. In this case, healing was complete within 2 weeks. The key to proper treatment of acute external otitis is in prevention and elimination of the cause. For swimmer's ear, offending water left in the ear canal is removed by the placement of 70% alcohol in the ear canal after swimming.

21

Chronic External Otitis

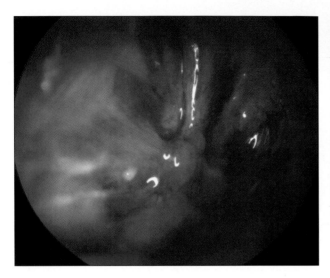

Fig 21–1

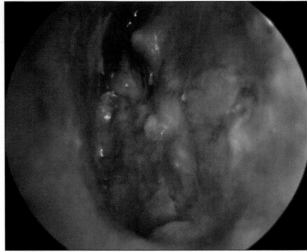

Fig 21–2

The otoscopic views are of a 35-year-old man with poor personal hygiene, with itchy ears and recurrent external otitis. Chronic external otitis is usually caused by the patient scratching the external ear canal because of a disturbing itch. The itch is of unknown etiology. Between episodes of infection, the ear canal may appear dry and scaly. The patient is urged not to scratch the ear or break the skin. Treatment must be continuous and can be from as little as daily flushing of the ear canal with 70% alcohol to as much as nightly installation of a steroid ointment in a Vaseline vehicle to prevent the itch. Whenever treatment is stopped, the itch will recur within a few days. This treatment can be used indefinitely.

22

Keratosis Obturans
(Cholesteatoma of the External
Auditory Canal)

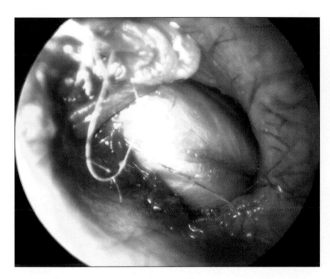

Fig 22–1

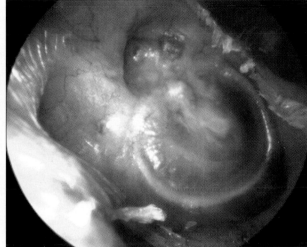

Fig 22–2

The otoscopic views are that of a right ear of a 58-year-old woman with normal hearing and chronic bronchitis. The otoscopic view on the left demonstrates a cholesteatoma mass filling the external auditory canal. Differential diagnosis could include: cholesteatoma debris from a mastoid cavity or encephalocele filling the ear canal from a mastoid cavity. The otoscopic view on the right demonstrates the same ear after the canal cholesteatoma was removed using a local anesthetic. The canal is extensively larger than normal with three depressions where normal bone has been absorbed, involving the floor of the external auditory canal lateral to the tympanic membrane annulus and one area in the posterior-superior quadrant, and another over the superior part exposing the head of the malleus and the epitympanum. Hearing was normal. The amount of bone destruction depends on the length of the time that the cholesteatoma is allowed to expand without treatment.[1] This type of cholesteatoma has an unknown cause and can be treated by regular observation and physical cleansing of the cholesteatoma from the external auditory canal or by surgical repair with the placement of cartilage or bone in the areas of erosion to reconstruct the external auditory canal. Considered observation and cleansing for a prolonged period is required.

Reference

1. Bunting WP. Ear canal cholesteatoma and bone absorption. *Trans Amer Acad Ophthal Otol.* 1968;72(2): 161–172.

23

Exostoses of the External Auditory Canal

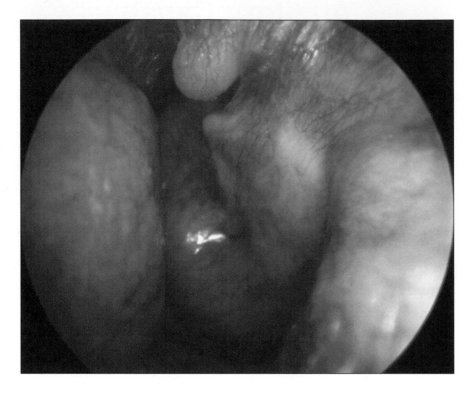

Fig 23–1

The physician often encounters exostoses during routine otoscopy. The lesions are asymptomatic and all that is required is that the examiner note their presence and tell the patient.[1] This is an otoscopic view of a left ear with a small exostoses anterior and lateral to the short process of the malleus and a larger one on the anterior wall of the external audi-tory canal appearing little different than a normal anterior canal wall bulge.

Reference

1. DiBartolomeo JR. Exostoses of the external auditory canal. *Ann Otol Rhinol Laryngol.* 1979;88(6, pt 2, suppl 61).

24

Nonobstructing Exostoses of the External Auditory Canal

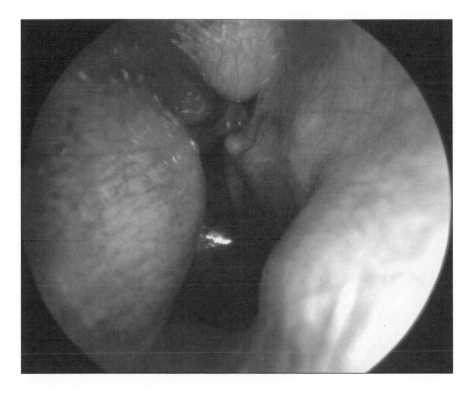

Fig 24–1

The otoscopic view is of a left ear with four nonobstructing exostoses. Exostoses of the external auditory canal are benign abnormal growths of bone that develop as semispherical masses beneath the skin of the external auditory canal and can produce obstruction. The condition is sometimes called "surfers ear" because exostoses tend to develop in people who swim in cold water. The masses are hard and painless. They are sessile and are usually multiple. Exostoses are to be distinguished from osteomas, which are usually solitary with a thin stalk or neck connecting them to the bone of the ear canal. No treatment is required unless symptoms of repeated otitis externa or frequent or inconvenient obstruction with debris or water develop. Characteristically, repeated exposure to cold water over a period of 20 years is required before obstruction develops. Rarely repeat removal is needed in patients with continuing exposure to cold water. Surgical removal usually involves restoration of the external auditory canal to its normal size with drills and curets by the transcanal approach through a speculum under local anesthesia as an outpatient procedure. Care must be taken to elevate and preserve the canal skin so that it can be replaced to obtain prompt healing and avoid stenosis. The operation can be extremely hazardous with risk of injury to the tympanic membrane, facial nerve, inner ear, and jugular bulb and requires that the surgeon have adequate training and experience in the management of this condition.

25

Nonobstructing Exostoses of the External Auditory Canal

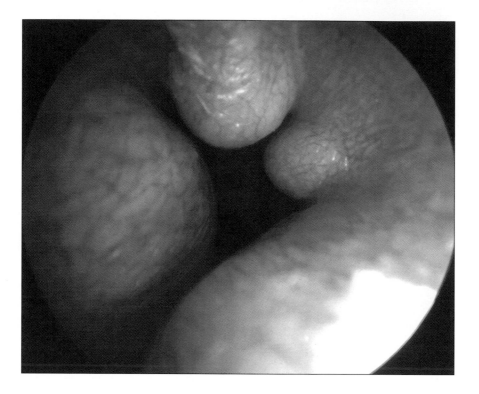

Fig 25–1

The otoscopic view is that of a left ear with four exostoses that are asymptomatic but are so large that obstruction could occur. A large exostosis protrudes from the posterior inferior external auditory canal and another large one from the anterior canal wall. A smaller exostosis involves the superior canal wall and the smallest involves the posterior superior canal wall. There is adequate space to admit a suction tip to aspirate debris.

Atlas of Otoscopy

26

Exostoses of the External Auditory Canal

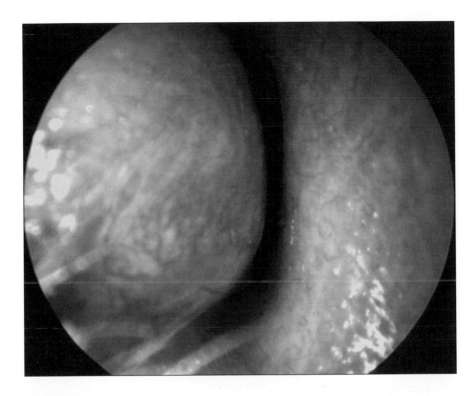

Fig 26–1

The otoscopic view is that of a left ear with a single, large globular sessile exostosis, almost completely obstructing the ear canal. Surgical approach is similar to that for canal skin tympanoplasty. Under a local or general anesthetic, the otologist, working through a speculum, makes an incision in the normal portion of the ear canal. The canal skin and periosteum is then elevated from the bone of the exostosis until there is no space for the instruments to move medially. The bone is then removed with a small drill or curette until space is again made to elevate more skin toward the annulus. This procedure is repeated by alternately removing bone and elevating skin and periosteum until the entire exostoses has been removed and the ear canal has a normal contour. Care is taken not to damage the canal skin with the drill or curette and the skin is left attached by a pedicle on its medial side. At the end of the procedure, the canal skin is placed over the newly contoured external auditory canal. The ear canal is filled with Gelfoam, soaked in an antibiotic aqueous steroid suspension to hold the pedicle skin flap against the bone. During bone removal, care should be taken to avoid exposing a large area of the glenoid fossa. Use of a postauricular incision for the treatment of exostoses offers no advantage other than giving a sense of false security to the inexperienced surgeon.

27

Exostoses Completely Obstructing the External Auditory Canal

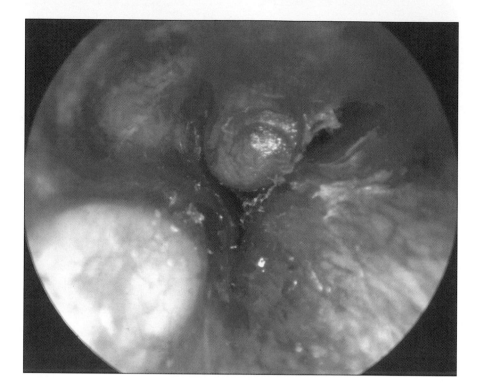

Fig 27–1

Three exostoses completely obstruct this right ear. The tympanic membrane cannot be seen. The opening will not admit a suction tip. The patient has pain and hearing loss from infection and retained debris medial to the obstructing masses. Prompt surgical removal of the exostoses is indicated.

SECTION IV

Acute Otitis Media

28

Viral Otitis Media

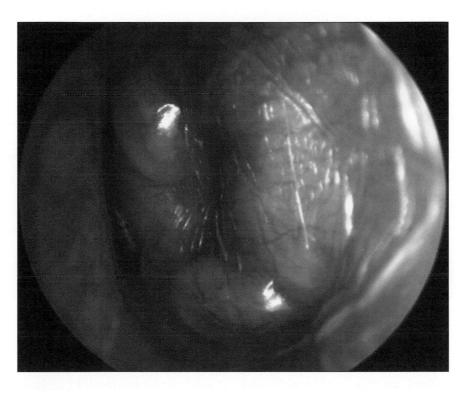

Fig 28–1

Viral otitis media is a frequent complication of the common cold. Serous otitis media may occur from Eustachian tube and Eustachian tube lymphatic obstruction of a cold but the virus in many cases may invade the mucosa of the tympanium to produce a secretory otitis media. A special form of viral otitis media involves the development of bullous myringitis. This condition is often complicated by the simultaneous invasion of the tympanum by hemolytic streptococci or pneumococci. This chapter demonstrates a view of the left tympanic membrane with bullous myringitis and exudate within the tympanum under pressure causing the pars tensa to bulge outward. Three blebs are seen on the anterior half of the pars tensa. Puncture of the blebs may be done to relieve pain. Viral otitis media may be associated with a simultaneous viral labyrinthitis with vertigo, sensorineural hearing loss, and tinnitus. Acute bacterial otitis media can be differentiated from an uncomplicated viral otitis media by the presence of fever and a positive culture that occur with the bacterial infection. Treatment for the latter type is with a systemic antibiotic and oral phenyl-propanylamine.

29

Bilateral Acute Suppurative Otitis Media: The Stage of Hyperemia

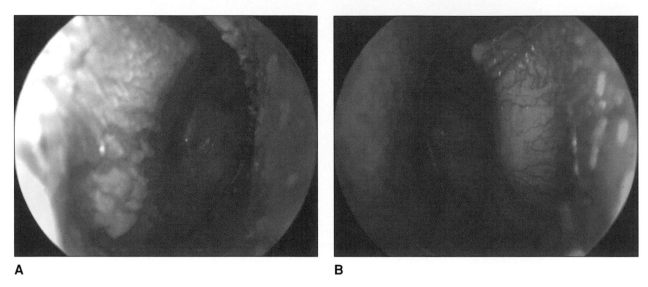

A   B

Fig 29–1. Otoscopic view of the right (A) and left (B) ears of a child with early suppurative otitis media.

The otoscopic views are those of the right and the left ears of a young patient with the first stage of acute suppurative otitis media. According to Shambaugh, the first reaction of the mucoperiosteum of the middle ear spaces to an invading microorganism is a simple hyperemia.[1] Otoscopy reveals loss of luster and injection of the vessels of the tympanic membrane but without enough thickening to cause loss of landmarks. The long and short process of the malleus is clearly seen on each side. Earache is usually present, accompanied by a sense of fullness. Fever is usually present and helps to differentiate a bacterial from a nonbacterial, viral, or sterile secretory otitis media. Hearing is usually nearly normal until fluid develops in the tympanum signaling a stage of exudation. For fulminating infections, which are most commonly due to beta-hemolytic streptococcus, an appropriate antibiotic should be given by injection. Milder infections are treated by oral antibiotics. Myringotomy is not useful in this stage. Local heat, analgesics, bed rest, and an effective oral decongestant such as phenylpropanolamine are useful.

Reference

1. Shambaugh, GE Jr. *Surgery of the Ear.* Philadelphia, Pa: W. B. Saunders; 1959:154.

30

Acute Suppurative Otitis Media: Stage of Exudation

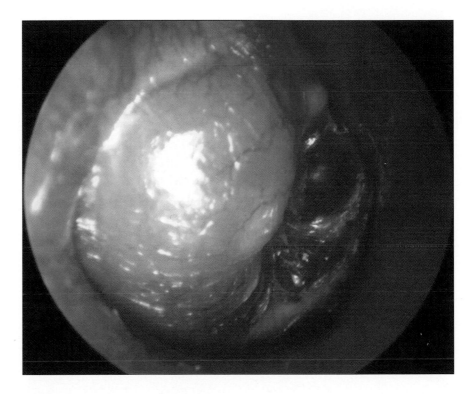

Fig 30–1

Shambaugh describes six stages of acute suppurative otitis media: (1) hyperemia, (2) exudation, (3) suppuration, (4) coalescence, (5) complication, and (6) resolution. This otoscopic view is of a right ear with acute suppurative otitis media in the stage of exudation. The entire posterior half of the pars tensa demonstrates the thickened bulging tympanic membrane with loss of landmarks. This portion appears pale and almost cream-colored instead of the usual red hyperemic appearance seen in the portion of the pars tensa anterior to the malleus and suggests that the organism is pneumococcus. The anterior half of the pars tensa has a series of several small bulges. The entire tympanic membrane and external auditory canal are hyperemic. The short process of the malleus can be seen near the center of the superior part of the annular ring. The middle ear and pneumatic cells are filled with exudate under pressure causing this otoscopic appearance. At this stage, there is usually increased pain and fever. Untreated, spontaneous rupture of the pars tensa and the development of the stage of suppuration usually occurs. If pain and toxicity are severe, immediate myringotomy to release the exudate under pressure is indicated. Prompt and intensive specific antibacterial therapy should be given with or without myringotomy.

31

Acute Suppurative Otitis Media: Late Stage of Exudation

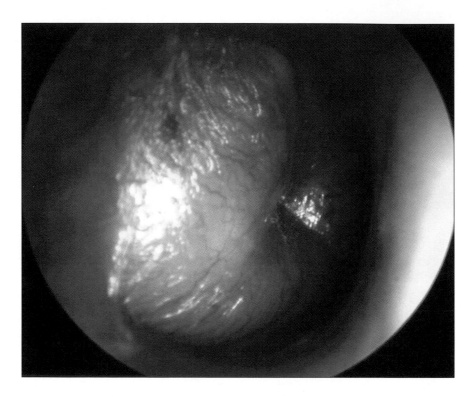

Fig 31–1

Acute suppurative otitis media with fever is of bacterial origin, most commonly caused by streptococcus and pneumococcus. Anything that interferes with the normal functioning of the Eustachian tubes including hypertrophied tonsils and adenoids, allergic edema of the Eustachian tube, viral salpingitis, and cleft palate predisposes one to an acute bacterial otitis media. This condition must be distinguished from sterile allergic and serous otitis media, viral otitis media, acute necrotic otitis media, tubercular chronic otitis media, and chronic (nontubercular) otitis media. There are six stages of acute otitis media: (1) hyperemia, (2) exudation, (3) suppuration, (4) coalescence, (5) complication, and (6) resolution. The otoscopic view of the right tympanic membrane demonstrates the state of exudation during which there is increased pain, fever, and toxicity. The pars tensa is thickened and bulges outward with loss of landmarks and light reflex. Red hyperemic arteries are seen crossing the vascular strip and toward the manubrium of the malleus. Exudate under pressure can be seen bulging the pars tensa inferior to the umbo. It is at this stage when accompanied with acute otalgia that a myringotomy is indicated to relieve the exudate under pressure. No anesthesia is necessary and relief is immediate. Without myringotomy spontaneous rupture may occur and lead to the same result. Appropriate systemic antibiotic treatment and oral phenylpropanolamine should be given until complete resolution has occurred.

32

Acute Otitis Media: Purulent Stage

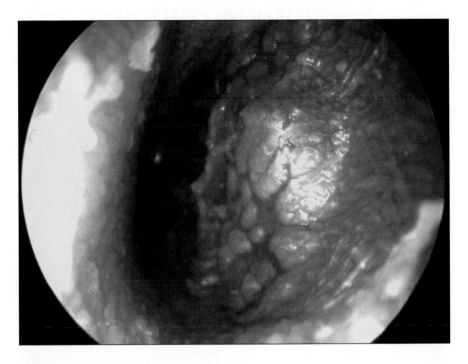

Fig 32–1

The otoscopic photograph shows a left ear in an advanced stage of acute otitis media. The posterior half of the pars tensa is bulging outward in an extreme position. The surface of the tympanic membrane has a pebbled appearance. The patient has severe otalgia and spontaneous rupture is imminent. When otalgia is present, myringotomy followed by appropriate antibiotic treatment is indicated. The myringotomy will provide instant relief of severe pain.

33

Acute Suppurative Otitis Media Following Spontaneous Tympanic Membrane Rupture

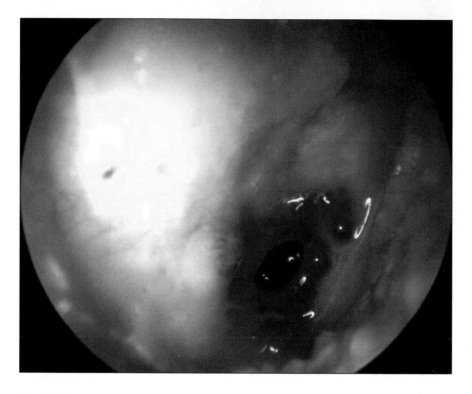

Fig 33–1

The otoscopic view is that of a left ear shortly after spontaneous rupture of the tympanic membrane. The tympanic membrane cannot be seen because the external auditory canal is filled with otorrhea of yellow pus and mucus. Although it is desirable to culture the pus before antibiotics are started, most such cases are treated empirically with systemic antibiotics. Resolution of the infection and the complete healing of the tympanic membrane is expected within 2 weeks. Follow-up visits for inspection of the tympanic membrane and to obtain a final audiogram are necessary to prevent relapse.

SECTION V

Disease of the Tympanic Membrane

34

Aerotitis

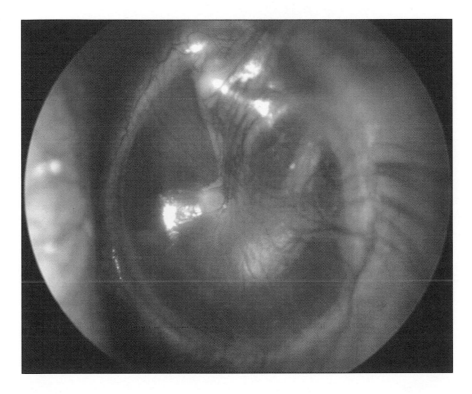

Fig 34–1

This is an otoscopic view of a left ear that shows evidence of barotrauma. The tympanic membrane appears to be completely normal with the exception of unusually prominent blood vessels along the long process of the malleus. There is no evidence of fluid in the middle ear, infection, or perforation. Hearing is usually normal. Barotrauma of this type is usually seen in air travelers who fly when they have a head cold or allergy. Typically the patient complains of pain in the ear during descent of the airplane from cruising altitude. In the absence of fluid or hearing loss, no treatment is necessary. More severe injury can result in ecchymosis along the long process of the malleus and serous otitis media. The condition usually resolves spontaneously within 3 weeks. Administration of oral phenylpropanolamine 50 mg four times daily (q.i.d.) and frequent performance of the Valsalva maneuver often speeds recovery. Myringotomy with insertion of a ventilating tube can be performed if the patient wishes to hear immediately.

35

Myringitis

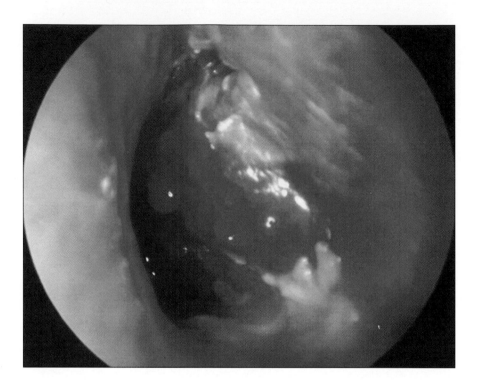

Fig 35–1

This is the otoscopic view of a left tympanic membrane with myringitis involvement. The central and posterior portions of the pars tensa are covered with florid granulation. The malleus is obscured. A white exudate is present at the inferior edge of the pars tensa and its junction with the floor of the external auditory canal. The uninvolved pars tensa is seen as a dark, semilunar area anteriorly. Superiorly, a small portion of the uninvolved pars flaccida is visible. Myringitis involves the squamous portion of the tympanic membrane and does not require the presence of a perforation or otitis media. The etiology may be bacterial, viral, or possibly allergy. A thorough understanding of this condition is not available. Treatment is topical in nature and involves intensive, prolonged administration of antibiotic and steroid-containing solutions. Uncontrolled granulating myringitis may persist for many years, resulting in the deposition of fibrous tissue lateral to the fibrous layers of the pars tensa, and eventual lateralization of the squamous epithelium at the meatus followed by eventual healing. Surgery for those cases involves removal of the fibrous core from the bony external auditory canal and fibrous pars tensa and placement of a skin graft into the normal position.

Epithelitis of a Tympanic Membrane Graft

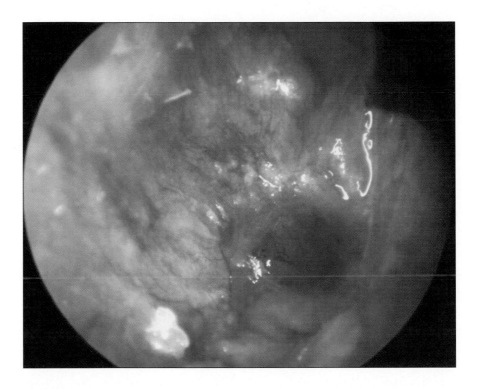

Fig 36–1

The otoscopic view of a left tympanic membrane graft involved with epithelitis is shown. Myringoplasty for the treatment of a dry central perforation had previously been performed with autogenous fascia as an onlay graft. The fascia had not been covered with canal skin. The tympanic membrane graft is intact. The otoscopic appearance, however, has an erythematous moist surface. Histologic examination of a cross section of a tympanic membrane so affected will demonstrate the presence of stratified squamous epithelium with a very thin cornified layer. The condition is called "epithelitis" and little is known about its cause. Although it can sometimes be troublesome, most cases have a benign course. Treatment involves the prolonged use of antibiotic corticosteroid ear drops topically. In rare cases the area must be excised and regrafted.

Chronic Granular Myringitis

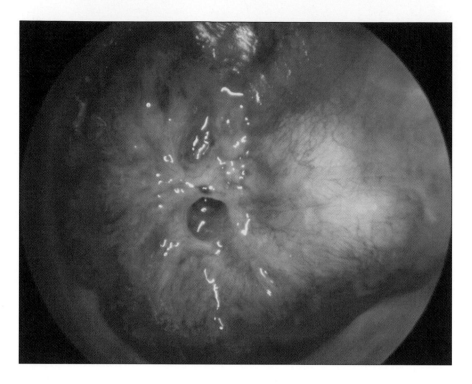

Fig 37–1

The otoscopic view shows a right ear. The anterior half of the pars tensa is covered by granulation tissue characteristic of chronic granular (granulating) myringitis. The anterior sulcus is obliterated by the granulation tissue. Chronic granular myringitis is among the rarer diseases of the ear and its etiology is unknown.[1] It has a painless course with symptoms of itching, otorrhea, and hearing loss. The inflammation is confined to the squamous layer of the tympanic membrane. It progresses over a period of weeks or months as a buildup of granulation tissue, after which the entire squamous epithelium melts away from the drum head. If untreated, over a period of 20 or 30 years the squamous epithelium may grow over the surface of the granulation, giving the appearance of a stenotic ear canal, with several millimeters of thick fibrous tissue between the normal fibrous layer of the tympanic membrane and the external skin. Persistent and prolonged treatment with anti-inflammatory antibiotic ear drops, systemic antibiotics, and local excision and cautery with 50% trichloracetic acid may effect a cure. Excision of the fibrous tissue or granulation from but not through the fibrous layer of the tympanic membrane and a graft of canal skin removed from the opposite ear may be required.

Reference

1. Pulec JL, Kinney SE. Diseases of the tympanic membrane. In: Paparella MM, Shumrick DA, eds. *Otolaryngology*. Vol 2. Philadelphia, Pa: W. B. Saunders Company; 1973:55–74.

38

The Atelectatic Ear

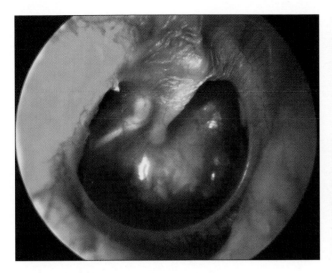

Fig 38–1. Atelectatic ear.

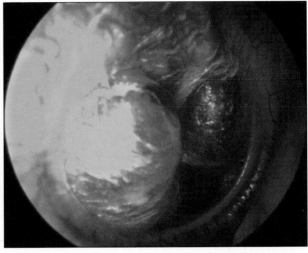

Fig 38–2. Atelectatic ear after inflation with Eustachian tube catheter.

The atelectatic ear is a specific and unique condition that produces conductive hearing loss. The otoscopic appearance is that of an intact, extremely thin, retracted pars tensa that is draped over the structures of the medial wall of the tympanum. The inexperienced observer may mistakenly think that there is a perforation. The pars flaccida is unaffected. The condition was well described by Richard Buckingham, who demonstrated that myringotomy and placement of a ventilating tube results in restoration of this thin membrane to its normal position within a few weeks and that the retraction would recur when the ventilating tube was removed. Buckingham erroneously attributed the problem to pathologic function of the Eustachian tube. In fact the pathology of the atelectatic ear is of the tympanic membrane and not of the Eustachian tube. It is caused either by an immune response or the results of suppurative otitis media, leading to loss of the middle fibrous layer of the tympanic membrane. The resulting two-layer tympanic membrane composed of squamous epithelium and mucous membrane does not have the tensile strength to resist the 4 cm of water vacuum that normally occurs between the periodic opening of the Eustachian

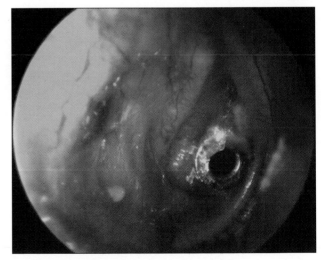

Fig 38–3. Atelectatic ear 6 weeks after installation of ventilating tubes.

tube. The thin membrane therefore moves into the tympanum. *No serous fluid develops.*

Treatment involves two steps. First, a ventilation tube is placed to prevent any vacuum from developing in the tympanum. The tube is usually placed over an air space in the tubotympanum. This allows the thin tympanic membrane to gradually detach itself from the ossicles and the promontory and return to the normal tense position. In some cases, there are areas of adhesive otitis as well, which do not become detached and require surgical dissection to repair. After the pars tensa has returned to its normal position, myringoplasty is performed to excise the pathologic tympanic membrane and replace it with a strong new graft that will withstand the normal vacuum of the tympanum. Homograft tympanic membranes are an ideal choice to replace the missing fibrous layer.

39

Atelectasis and Serous Otitis Media

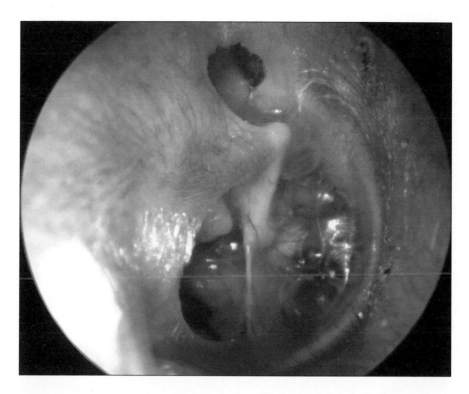

Fig 39–1

The otoscopic view is that of a right ear with both atelectasis and serous fluid. These are two separate, *unrelated* coexisting conditions. Amber serous fluid and air bubbles can be seen through the retracted intact two-layered anterior half of the pars tensa anterior to the vertical manubrium of the malleus. The lenticular process of the incus and round window niche are seen through the retracted posterior half of the pars tensa. The retraction extends beyond the view posterior to the annulus. The pars flaccida is retracted into an enlarged notch of Rivinus. The presence of air bubbles suggests that the serous fluid is transitory. It is not possible to determine if there is only atelectasis or also adhesive otitis media without inflation. See Chapter 38.

40

Atelectasis and Serous Otitis Media (Postinflation)

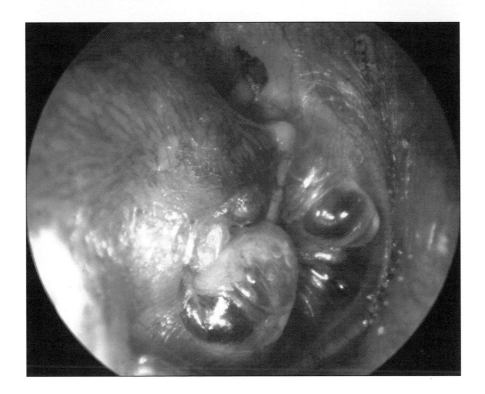

Fig 40–1

This is the same ear shown in Chapter 39. The photograph demonstrates the result of middle-ear inflation by the Valsalva maneuver. The posterior very thin but intact pars tensa retraction is seen protruding into the external auditory canal. There are no adhesions of the membrane to the structures of the tympanum. Treatment is myringoplasty performed through the external auditory canal through a speculum.[1] A strong new graft is capable of withstanding the normal vacuum of 3 cm of water in the tympanum.

Reference

1. Pulec JL, Kinney SE. Diseases of the tympanic membrante. In: Paparella MM, Shumrick DA, eds. *Otolaryngology*. Vol 2. Philadelphia, Pa: W. B. Saunders Company; 1973:55–74.

SECTION VI

Serous Otitis Media

41

Serous Otitis Media

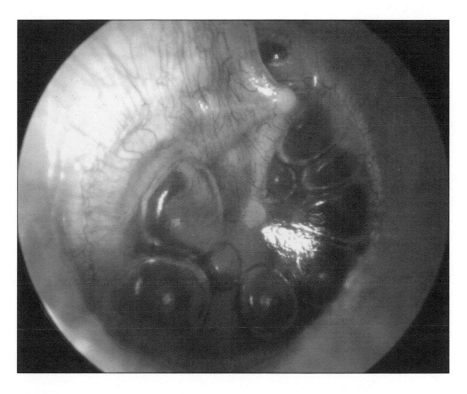

Fig 41–1

Fluid behind the tympanic membrane with or without the presence of air bubbles is a common cause for conductive hearing loss. The otoscopic appearance is that of an intact tympanic membrane with an amber dull appearance. There are several variations in appearance and in the etiology and pathogenesis of the fluid. The condition may be overlooked by an inexperienced physician. Use of the operating microscope might be necessary to adequately see the pathologic changes. Clinical diagnosis is easy when air can be forced into the tympanum by the Valsalva maneuver or by the use of the Eustachian tube catheter and listening tube. The presence of air bubbles or the meniscus of a fluid level is pathogonomic of serous otitis media. Treatment is directed toward the cause.

Summary of mechanisms of production of serous otitis media[1]:

A. Eustachian tube lumen obstruction
  1. Direct obstruction by
    a. Fracture
    b. Hypertrophic tonsils and adenoids
    c. Polyp or neoplasm
  2. Mucosal edema from allergy or inflammation
  3. Piston effect of ciliary action on a mucous plug
B. Obstruction of Eustachian tubal lymphatics[2]
  1. Inflammation
    a. Infected tonsils and adenoids
    b. Sinusitis
  2. Nasopharyngeal tumor
  3. Radiation
  4. Allergy
C. Middle ear effusion without vacuum
  1. Allergy
  2. Viral infection
  3. Cholesterol granuloma

References

1. Pulec JL, Horwitz MJ. Diseases of the Eustachian tube. In: Paparella MM, Shumrick DA, eds. *Otolaryngology.* Vol 2. Philadelphia, Pa: W. B. Saunders Company; 1973:75–92.

2. Pulec JL, Kamio T, Graham MD. Eustachian tube lymphatics. *Ann Otol Rhinol Laryngol.* 1975;84(4):483–492.

42

Serous Otitis Media With Retraction of the Pars Tensa

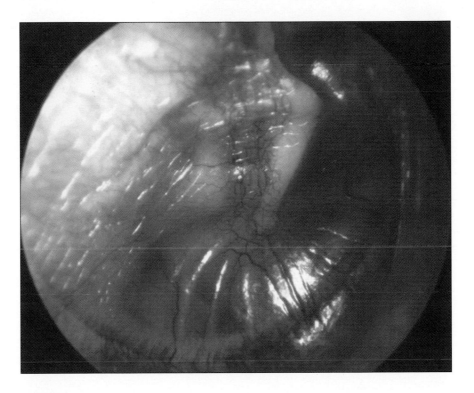

Fig 42–1

The otoscopic view is of a right ear with serous otitis media. The entire pars tensa is slightly retracted. The most evident retraction is seen anteriorly where the annulus seems to protrude because of the inward position of the pars tensa. The dull amber appearance is indicative of serous otitis media.

Treatment is directed to the etiology such as allergy, sinus infection, or hypertrophied tonsils and adenoids. Serous otitis media present more than 3 weeks without spontaneous resolution can be treated with myringotomy, aspiration of the serous fluid, and the placement of a ventilating tube.

43

Secretory Otitis Media (Glue Ear)

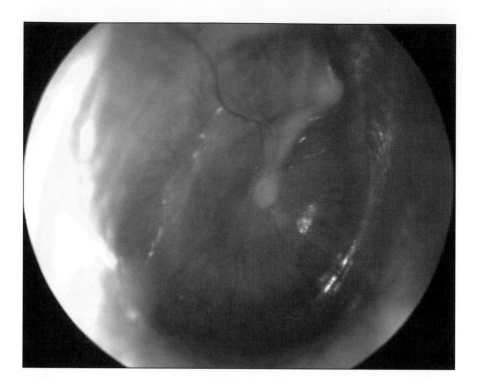

Fig 43–1

Although secretory otitis media in which the tympanum is filled with gluelike material has many of the clinical features of serous otitis media, the etiology, otoscopic appearance, and clinical course are different. As in serous otitis media pneumatic otoscopy reveals reduced mobility of the tympanic membrane. The golden brown caramel color seen through the translucent drum suggests the presence of glue and is often diagnostic of secretory otitis media. The dull surface appears to have a slight bulge rather than a normal or retracted appearance. "Glue ear" is most common between the ages of 3 and 6 years and is seldom seen after adolescence. Myringotomy with insertion of a ventilating button is the treatment of choice. The thick tenacious clear colored elastic material has the characteristics of rubber cement and can often be stretched to a strand 2 or 3 inches long before a volume can be extracted from the tympanum using a suction tip. The gluelike mucous material is similar to that sometimes seen in the nose after a specific viral infection and is most likely the result of a similar viral infection of the goblet cells of the membrane of the middle ear.

44

Serous Otitis Media With Tympanosclerosis and Healed Neomembrane

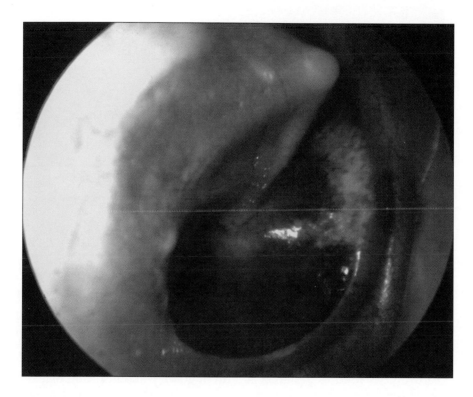

Fig 44–1

It is common for ears with abnormal appearance and evidence of previous disease to function normally and be trouble-free. The otoscopic view is that of a right ear with an acute episode of serous otitis media. The short process of the malleus at the superior edge of the photograph is dominant. The handle of the malleus is intact and retracted. The pars flaccida appears completely normal. The pars tensa is intact but the majority has had a large central perforation and is replaced with a thin neomembrane. The yellow fluid of serous otitis media gives the tympanic membrane a dull amber appearance. At the anterior inferior edge of the healed perforation, a small air bubble can be seen within the tympanum. The three-layered portion of the pars tensa remains as a ring approximately 2 mm wide, extending inferiorly from the pars flaccida in the superior-anterior part of the photograph to the posterior-inferior portion where it widens to demonstrate preservation of most of the posterior-superior part of the pars tensa. A small area of tympanosclerosis 3 mm wide involves the anterior-superior quadrant of the pars tensa. A light reflex can be seen anterior to the umbo in the center of the photograph and also in the area of the air bubble. Treatment for this ear is conservative, with oral antihistamine and phenylpropanolamine decongestant and the frequent use of the Valsalva maneuver.

45

Blue Eardrum

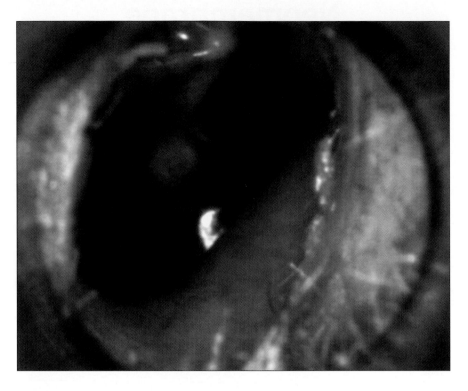

Fig 45–1

The term "blue eardrum" is used to designate a specific type of serous otitis media in which the fluid contains hemosiderin from disintegrating red cells, usually originating from cholesterol granuloma. The otoscopic view of the tympanic membrane reveals a dull, bluish color which is usually not as dark or black in appearance as hemotympanum. The history is similar to that of serous otitis media and the treatment is similar. Allergy is often a prominent factor and it is not uncommon for a profuse exudative discharge to develop after myringotomy and insertion of a ventilating tube. In such a case treatment is local and must be persistent with eardrops that are forced through the ear and down the Eustachian tube four times daily (q.i.d.). A medication found to be an effective ear drop for this condition is gamma globulin (suitable for injection intramuscularly) and Vasocidin a.a., Sig: gtts. ii q.i.d. Mastoid surgery is usually not indicated and should be considered only as a last resort after months of persistent conservative treatment.

46

Blue Eardrum and Cholesterol Granuloma

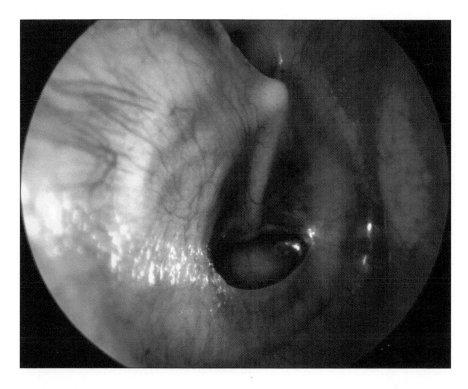

Fig 46–1

The otoscopic view is that of a right ear. The short process of the malleus is at the center of the top of the photo. Extending immediately downward from this is the long process of the malleus. Inferior to the umbo a neomembrane is retracted against the promontory, which appears as a yellowish globular mass. There is a scar involving the posterior and inferior edge of the pars tensa. The entire tympanic membrane appears blue and has been described as a "blue eardrum." This condition is to be distinguished from hemotympanum, which represents blood within the tympanum. In this case, the patient has cholesterol granuloma which is frequently associated with serous otitis media. Disintegrating red blood cells in the serous fluid give the blue color to the tympanic membrane. Initial treatment is to do a myringotomy and place a ventilating tube. Any profuse mucous otorrhea is treated with an eardrop of equal parts Vasocidin and gamma globulin. If after weeks of persistent local treatment, otorrhea persists, a surgical toilette of mastoid and middle ear can be performed to help resolve the process. Patience and persistent treatment are required to resolve this subacute type of otitis media.

47

Cholesterol Granuloma

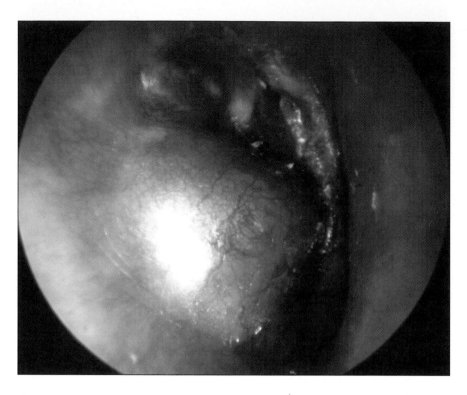

Fig 47–1

The otoscopic view of a left ear is similar to that of a "blue eardrum" with the addition of a yellowish spot caused by tissue in the tympanum touching the tympanic membrane. This appearance is typical of cholesterol granuloma with serous otitis media. The condition is caused by infection and or allergic formation of masses of granulation tissue within the middle ear and mastoid. The patient's immune system is able to control the bacterial infection but complete resolution to normal does not occur.

Treatment involves myringotomy with insertion of a ventilating tube and instillation of an antibiotic steroid eardrop with an aqueous vehicle. Should resolution not occur, with conservative treatment, a Pulec type V tympanoplasty to establish drainage from the mastoid to the Eustachian tube through the facial recess without disturbing the bony external auditory canal or the attic or ossicular chain will usually solve the problem.

48

Extensive Cholesterol Granuloma

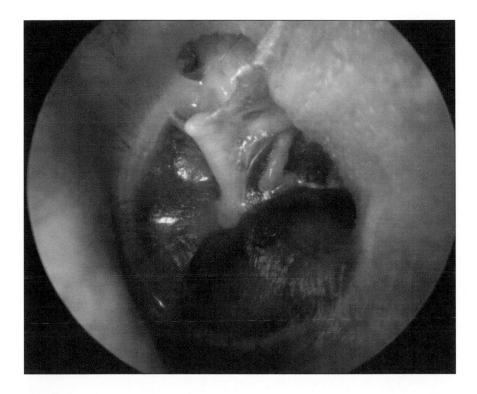

Fig 48–1

The otoscopic view is that of a left ear with an intact tympanic membrane, obvious serous otitis media, tympanosclerosis of the pars tensa, and a mass behind the posterior superior quadrant of the pars tensa causing the membrane to bulge. This is a mass of cholesterol granuloma secondary to unresolved infection or allergy. It is not possible to exclude neoplasm, and for that reason, surgical removal, the establishment of a diagnosis, and drainage of the mastoid and middle ear are indicated. The procedure of choice is the Pulec type V tympanoplasty, which involves complete mastoidectomy and the opening of the facial recess without disturbing the tympanic membrane, external auditory canal, the ossicular chain, or the attic. Following this procedure the conductive hearing loss resolves within 4 weeks. Should a neoplasm be found by frozen section histopathologic examination, the operative procedure can be modified accordingly.

49

Grommet Ventilation Myringostomy

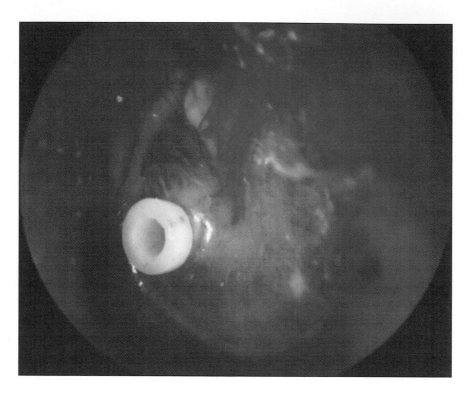

Fig 49–1

Grommet ventilation myringostomy illustrated is the typical appearance of a Teflon grommet within a myringotomy incision. A myringotomy incision will become closed within several hours. Whenever chronic ventilation is required, a tube of some sort must be placed through the myringotomy opening to keep it patent. The majority of patients are cooperative and the procedure is performed in the office with the use of anesthesia by a single injection of Xylocaine or by Iontophoresis. The actual myringotomy and insertion of the grommet is a 60-second procedure. Performed by a trained otologist using the operating microscope, the myringotomy can be performed anywhere on the pars tensa without injury to the chorda tympani, ossicular chain, or round window. The nature of the condition being treated dictates the position for the myringotomy. Ideally the myringotomy incision is made halfway between the umbo and the annulus, perpendicular to and centered on a line that passes through the long process of the malleus. Grommets are manufactured from a variety of different metal and plastic materials. Only those made of Silastic are known to cause an allergic reaction with granulation tissue growth around the tube in a small percentage of cases. The presence of a grommet causes an imperceptible 4-dB conductive hearing loss. The grommet is spontaneously extruded after about 4 months in small children and in adults may remain in place for 1–5 years.

Atlas of Otoscopy

50

Blue Silastic Grommet Ventilating Tube

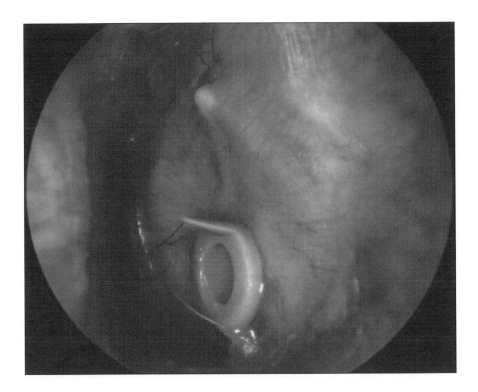

Fig 50–1

A variety of commercially available ventilating tubes and grommets have been devised for the treatment of serous otitis media. The photograph represents the otoscopic view of a left tympanic membrane with a blue Silastic grommet maintaining an opening through the tympanic membrane. The ear is dry and there is no evidence of serous fluid. The blue button has a tongue at its superior edge, which could be used to extract it with a cup forceps or alligator forceps. The grommet is in position inferior to the umbo, halfway between the umbo and the annulus and in line with the long process of the malleus. This ventilating tube is in a correct position and has no evidence of inflammation. Tubes made of Silastic tend to be less delicately made than tubes made with stiffer material. A small percentage of patients are allergic to Silastic and develop reactive granulation tissue around the grommet. Should a reaction develop, treatment involves simple removal of the grommet and instillation of an ear drop containing an antibiotic and steroid. One reason the tube is colored blue may be to make it more obvious to the less experienced physician who might look into the ear.

51

Small Blue Grommet Ventilating Tube

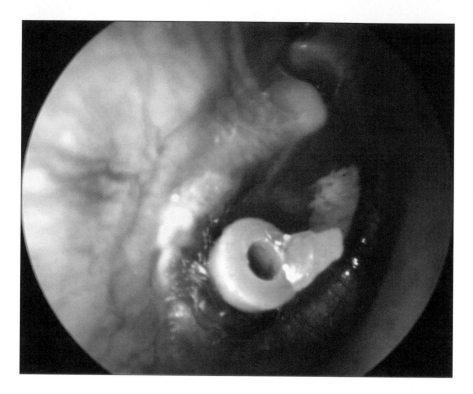

Fig 51–1

The otoscopic view is that of a right ear with a blue Silastic grommet at the lower center of the photograph. The middle ear had been filled with mucus. The true nature of the etiology and pathogenesis of all varieties of fluid within the middle ear is not completely understood, although the viscid mucous-type of fluid is usually caused by an immunologic process. The most common form in children is due to cows' milk allergy. Placement of this grommet is excellent and the tympanic membrane is now in the normal position. The grommet has a small-caliber opening and a protrusion extending outward designed to make extraction easy. The protrusion can be grasped by a cup or alligator forceps and removed. A small patch of white tympanosclerosis is in the anterior part of the pars tensa. To the left of the grommet is a brownish, cream-colored dry secretion. Anterior to the neck of the malleus the pars flaccida is retracted but all of the surface is visible.

52

Long-term Ventilation Myringostomy

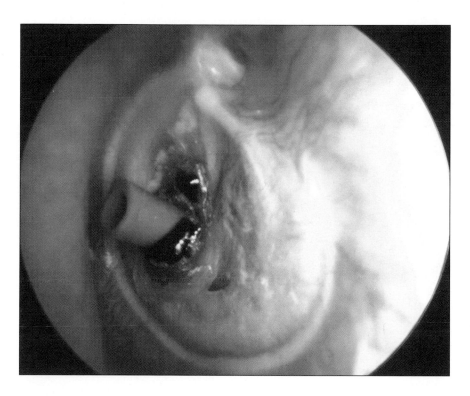

Fig 52–1

This photograph shows a green Silastic T-shaped tube protruding through the myringotomy immediately anterior and inferior to the umbo of a left tympanic membrane. A spot of ebony-colored dried blood lies inferior to the tube adjacent to the tympanic membrane. A small spot of dried blood lies superior and posterior to the tube. The tube is open and the tympanum is well aerated. Several small flecks of tympanosclerosis are seen lying within the tympanic membrane both anterior and posterior to malleus. A 1 × 2 mm, more translucent two-layer part of the tympanic membrane devoid of the medial fibrous layer is seen immediately posterior and inferior to the umbo. The pars flaccida is slightly retracted. A variety of tubes with a very large flange or mesh disk within the middle ear has been designed to help prevent extrusion with long-term use. The first tube of this type was designed by John Per-Lee. Tubes of this type are designed to stay in place for several years for patients with long-lasting problems such as serous otitis media with cleft palate. Since 4 or 5% of patients develop a Silastic allergy, it is probably best to use tubes made of other materials. An allergic response results in the development of florid granulation tissue from the tympanic membrane in contact with and surrounding the tube.

53

Ventilating Tube in an Atelectatic Ear

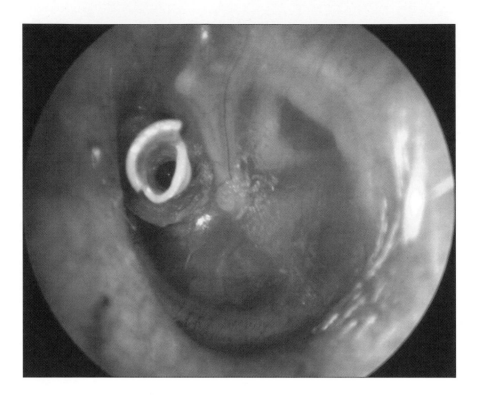

Fig 53–1

The accompanying otoscopic view shows a left ear with a ventilating tube through the anterior superior quadrant of the tympanic membrane. This is a case of an atelectatic ear, in which the tympanic membrane was retracted over the ossicular chain and promontory, so that the only space containing air was the tubotympanum. Myringotomy and placement of the tube were performed 6 weeks before this photograph was taken. The thin, retracted pars tensa naturally returned to its normal position within 3 weeks. Removal of the tube with healing of the pars tensa would likely result in a prompt recurrence of the atelectasis.

The atelectatic tympanic membrane is *not* a problem of the Eustachian tube[1] but is a result of loss of the fibrous layer of the pars tensa. Definitive treat-

ment involves surgical removal of the damaged tympanic membrane and replacement with a strong fibrous material, such as a homograft tympanic membrane or fascia or perichondrium. The real problem is that the weakened pars tensa cannot withstand the 4 cm of water vacuum that normally occurs before the normal, periodic opening of the Eustachian tube. The etiology is a loss of the fibrous layer through an immune response or to acute necrotizing otitis media.

Reference

1. Pulec JL, Kinney SE. Diseases of the tympanic membrane. In: Paparella MM, Shumrick DA, eds. *Otolaryngology*. Vol 2. Philadelphia, Pa: W. B. Saunders Company; 1973:55–74.

54

Grommet Placement Over Tubotympanum

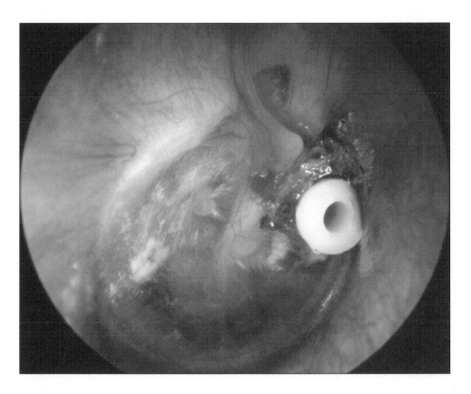

Fig 54–1

The otoscopic view is that of a right ear that was atelectatic before myringotomy. The entire pars tensa was adherent to the media wall of the middle ear with the exception of a small air-containing space over the tubotympanum in the anterior superior quadrant. In this case, the Teflon grommet that appears as a white button in the right center of the photograph was placed in this only air-containing portion of the middle ear. The pars tensa has returned to its normal tense position and at this time appears normal with the exception of a small amount of white patchy tympanosclerosis in the posterior superior quadrant of the pars tensa. There is no serous otitis media. Anterior to the neck of the malleus, the pars flaccida is retracted but the entire surface is visible and requires no treatment at this stage. Dried secretion is seen superior to the Teflon button. Placement of grommets in this position can sometimes be technically difficult if the ear canal is very small or there is a large anterior canal wall bulge. Long-term treatment requires permanent use of a ventilating tube or preferably myringoplasty with the construction of a strong tympanic membrane that will withstand the normal vacuum of −4 mm of water.

55

Metallic Grommet Ventilating Tube

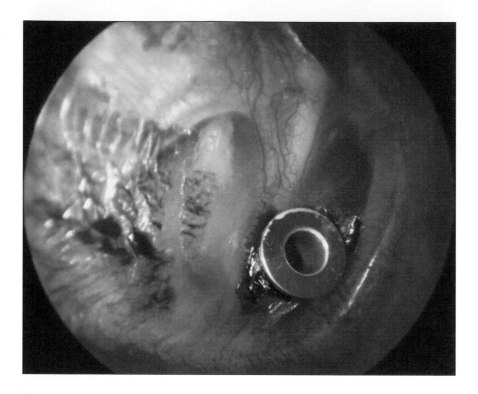

Fig 55–1

The otoscopic view is that of a right ear with a metallic grommet placed through a myringotomy inferior to the umbo. Dried blood is covering the surface of the metallic grommet and surrounds it near the myringotomy opening. The posterior canal wall and posterior part of the pars tensa is also stained with dried blood. The pars tensa is expanded into its normal position and there is no fluid within the middle ear. The incus and stapes can be seen through the tympanic membrane in the poste-rior superior quadrant. A variety of metals is used including titanium and gold. Use of a metallic tube is at the discretion of the surgeon and metallic tubes are equally as effective as other types. No allergic reaction has been noted. Metallic tubes tend to be more expensive than other types. Technically, the metallic tube is slightly more difficult to insert because the hard surface prevents the surgeon from being able to use a sharp needle against the rim to place the button into the myringotomy opening.

56

Large Green Silastic Grommet

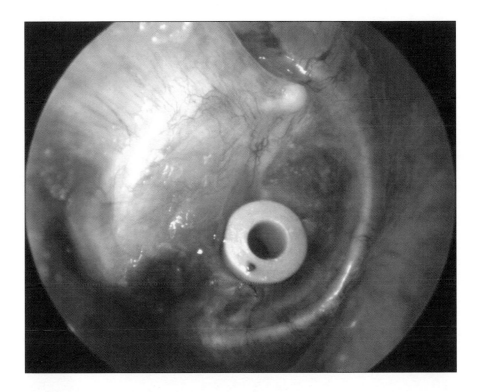

Fig 56–1

The otoscopic view is that of a right ear demonstrating a green Silastic grommet within a myringotomy. Immediately inferior to the umbo, the short process of the malleus protrudes from the tympanic membrane at the superior edge of the photograph and appears as a cream-colored globular protrusion. The placement of the tube is excellent and there is no evidence of serous otitis media. At the left edge of the photograph a brownish discoloration of dried blood from the initial procedure is seen. The green Silastic button has a large central opening. Anterior to the neck of the malleus the pars flaccida is retracted but all areas are visible.

57

Long-term Ventilating Tube With Tympanosclerosis

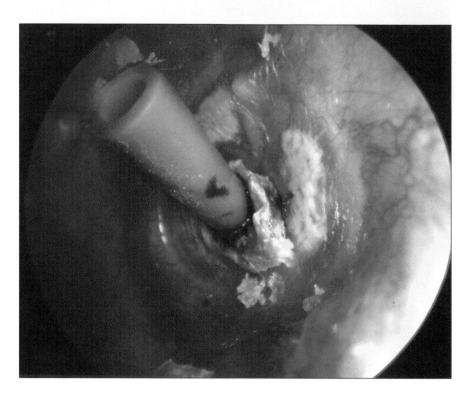

Fig 57–1

The otoscopic view is that of a left ear with a green Silastic ventilation tube in a myringotomy. The green tube demonstrates one problem that can occur with the long tube. The end of the tube is touching the anterior canal wall and can cause irritation, discomfort, and sometimes obstruction. It is sometimes necessary to cut the end of the tube to prevent it from touching the ear canal. Small patches of tympanosclerosis of a cosmetic type are anterior to the malleus and in the posterior half of the tympanic membrane. A crust is seen around the tube near the pars tensa and is not uncommonly seen when tubes are in place for long periods of time. Use of a long-term ventilating myringostomy tube is commonly necessary in patients who have persisting serous otitis media in association with a cleft palate.

58

Reaction From Long-term Ventilating Tube

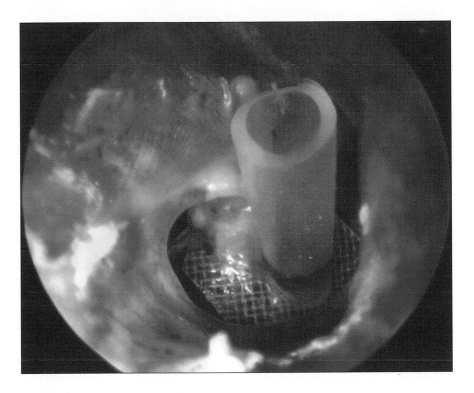

Fig 58–1

The otoscopic view shows a right ear in which a ventilating tube has been in place for over 2 years. There is evidence of chronic inflammation and pus. The pars tensa is injected from inflammation. A 30% central perforation of the pars tensa represents the enlargement of the original myringotomy opening. Within the tympanum and perforation is a Silastic mesh tube designed for long-term use. In the adult, tubes of this type can last indefinitely without diffi-

culty. In children, however, it is not uncommon to see the development of granulation tissue and enlargement of the myringotomy anytime after being in place for more than 1 year. In the case pictured above, there is no longer a reason to leave the ventilating tube in the ear and it should be removed. The resulting perforation can be left untreated until the surgeon feels comfortable that serous fluid will not return. Myringoplasty is necessary to repair the ear.

59

Ventilating Tube With Otitis Media

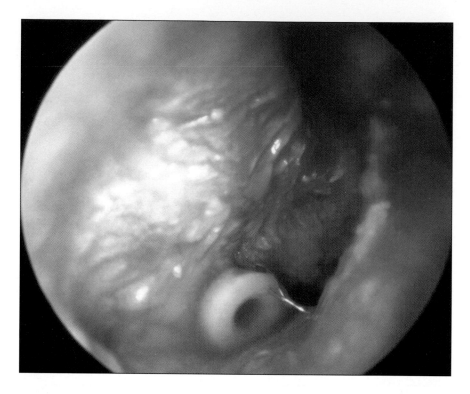

Fig 59–1

This is an otoscopic view of a right ear with a green Silastic ventilating tube and a removal wire through a myringotomy inferior to the umbo and very near the inferior annulus. Mucopus can be seen exuding through the ventilating tube. The entire pars tensa is thick and inflamed and gives the appearance of having fluid in the tympanum. This is a typical appearance of a ventilating tube in an ear that has become secondarily infected. This is not an uncommon occurrence, especially in children. Although an upper respiratory infection or cold can be the cause of acute otitis media in an ear that otherwise has been dry, the most usual cause in children is that they get water in the ear during swimming or bathing. Although some physicians allow their patients with ventilating tubes to swim, many episodes of ear infections can be avoided if the child does not swim and care is taken to keep water out of the ear. When otorrhea does occur, treatment is by both systemic antibiotics and the use of ear drops containing antibiotics and steroids. Treatment, in general, also may include avoidance of all cow's milk products, identification of specific offending allergens, and the performance of a complete tonsillectomy and adenoidectomy.

60

Perforation After Grommet Insertion

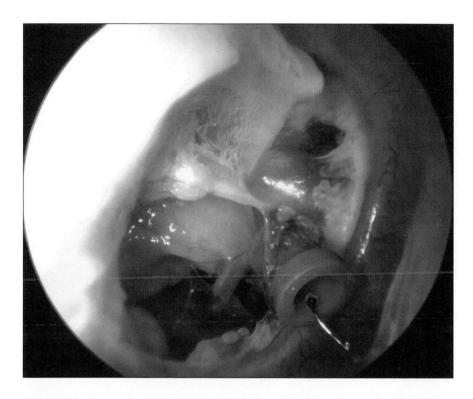

Fig 60–1

The otoscopic view is that of a right ear with a blue Silastic grommet ventilating tube in a myringotomy within the anterior edge of the pars tensa. Immediately to the left of the grommet is a 50% dry central perforation that occurred after an infection following the grommet insertion and despite insertion of the grommet. Perforations of this type are usually caused by beta-hemolytic streptococcus, which typically produces acute necrotizing otitis media. The superior part of the pars tensa is intact and the handle of the malleus and incus and stapes can be seen through the translucent membrane. The long process of the incus appears to be partially eroded. Through the perforation the media wall of the tympanum is seen containing the round window niche and the crevices in the hypotympanum. At the inferior edge of the perforation are two, small dry yellow masses that represent granulation tissue. The grommet contains a wire that can be used for extraction. Surgical repair by myringoplasty is not indicated until the cause of the recurrent fluid or recurrent infection has been solved. Treatment may involve the elimination of chronic sinusitis, avoidance of or desensitization to offending allergens, repair of a cleft palate, treatment of agammaglobulinemia or tonsillectomy and adenoidectomy.

61

Grommet Ventilation Myringostomy With Cholesteatoma

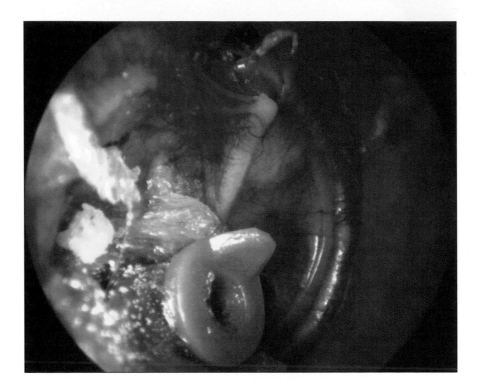

Fig 61–1

The otoscopic view is that of a right ear with a green Silastic grommet in proper position inferior to the umbo. Notably an attic cholesteatoma is evident at the superior edge of the photo and cholesteatoma in the posterior half of the tympanic membrane. Use of a grommet in an ear of this type cannot be expected to be useful in preventing progression or causing improvement in the disease. An ear of this type requires definitive surgery with removal of the cholesteatoma, aeration of the tympanum, and graft of the tympanic membrane. After such a procedure has been accomplished, use of a ventilating tube might then be indicated to treat any persisting serous otitis media. Some surgeons routinely perform a myringotomy and place a ventilating tube in the pars tensa after all tympanoplasty and mastoidectomy procedures. The authors do not advise this approach.

SECTION VII

Chronic Suppurative Otitis Media

62

Classification of Chronic Suppurative Otitis Media

We have developed and recommend a classification for chronic suppurative otitis media that includes six different types of pathologic involvement, in addition to a normal ear and one with complications such as brain abscess or meningitis, labyrinthine fistula, labyrinthitis, venous thrombosis, facial paralysis, encephalocele, and cerebrospinal fluid otorrhea. The classification is determined primarily by otoscopic examination of the tympanic membrane and ear canal but is augmented by patient history and other physical tests.

Classification

Type I: Perforation of the Tympanic Membrane Alone Without Evidence of Other Disease

A dry central perforation of the pars tensa may be as small as a pinhole or it may be so total that all that remains is the fibrous annulus (Fig 62–1A). Ears in this category have no squamous epithelium within the tympanum or mastoid, the ossicular chain is intact and mobile, and hearing loss is related to the size of the perforation. Ears of this type characteristically remain dry and trouble-free with the exception of hearing loss until water enters the tympanum or the patient develops an upper respiratory infection or allergy. Painless otorrhea usually follows contamination with water and upper respiratory infection of allergic exacerbation. Treatment with the appropriate systemic antibiotics and topical antibiotic steroid suspension results in the ear becoming dry within 2 weeks. The ear remains dry until the patient sustains another similar event. This process of repeated isolated periods of otorrhea followed by long periods without drainage is characteristic. A subvariety is the atelectatic ear, which has an absent fibrous layer of the pars tensa and intact squamous and mucous membrane layers. Treatment involves reconstructing the pars tensa for the purpose of restoration of hearing and prevention of recurrent otorrhea.

Type II: Conductive Hearing Loss With Intact Tympanic Membrane

Chronic otitis media can cause fixation or destruction of the ossicular chain with subsequent healing of the tympanic membrane (Fig 62–1B). In this category, the ear is dry, free from infection, and the tympanic membrane is intact. The major problem is that of hearing loss. The conductive hearing loss may be caused by fixation of the ossicular chain by a congenital fixation of bone, by tympanosclerosis involving the ossicular chain, fracture or dislocation of the ossicular chain from trauma, or dissolution of part of the ossicular chain from infection or immunologic effects.

Treatment is directed to restoration of hearing. Ossicular reconstruction and middle ear work can be performed through a tympanomeatal flap similar to that required for a stapedectomy.

Type III: Tympanic Membrane Perforation With Disease Confined to the Middle Ear and Epitympanum

This category involves a combination of type I and type II with the addition of the possibility of cholesteatoma and squamous epithelium involving the tympanic cavity (Fig 62–1C). There may be a central perforation with squamous epithelium extending onto the medial surface of the pars tensa or the squamous epithelium may extend over the promontory and seal off the tubotympanum. This category includes forms of adhesive otitis media in which the tympanic membrane is retracted and adherent to the promontory. The goal of treatment is not only to restore hearing but also to eliminate infection and to reconstruct the tympanic membrane.

Type IV: Attic Cholesteatoma

Attic cholesteatoma develops as expanding herniation of the pars flaccida into the epitympanum, mastoid, and middle ear (Fig 62–1D). Except in the most advanced cases, the pars tensa is uninvolved. This type of cholesteatoma usually remains dry and

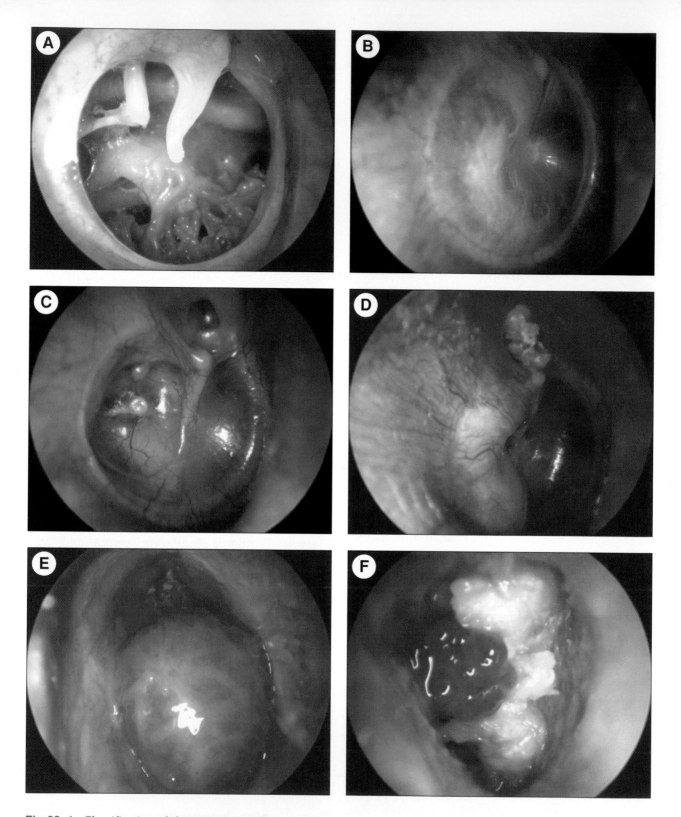

Fig 62–1. Classification of chronic otitis media.

A. Type I. Dry perforation of the tympanic membrane involving only the pars tensa. The ossicular chain is intact. The tympanum is free from disease.

B. Type II. Intact tympanic membrane with minimal tympanosclerosis. Conductive hearing loss caused by fixation of the stapes by tympanosclerosis.

C. Type III. Tympanic membrane perforation with disease confined to the middle ear and epitympanum. Tympanosclerosis is seen in the anterior pars tensa remnant. The posterior two thirds of the pars tensa perforation is healed with a neomembrane, which is retracted onto the promontory. The lenticular process of the incus has been eroded and the stapes head can be seen through the neomembrane.

D. **Type IV.** Attic cholesteatoma. A perforation is seen involving the pars flaccida anterior to the malleus. The pars tensa is intact. A cream-colored cholesteatoma sac is seen pressing against the medial surface of the pars tensa in the posterior superior one third of the tympanum.

E. **Type V.** Disease involving the middle ear, epitympanum, and mastoid without cholesteatoma. A large raspberry-colored granulation tissue polyp extending through a perforation of the pars tensa fills three quarters of the external auditory canal. There is purulent drainage with no evidence of cholesteatoma.

F. **Type VI.** Disease involving the middle ear, epitympanum, and mastoid with cholesteatoma. This otoscopic view shows silvery-white cholesteatoma debris and a granulation tissue polyp coexisting in the external auditory canal and extending through the pars tensa perforation. This is the most severe form of this disease.[1]

free of drainage unless the cholesteatomatous debris becomes wet and infected. Its development is insidious, with a progressive conductive hearing loss and eventually the development of a labyrinthine fistula or facial paralysis. This condition is significantly different from chronic suppurative otitis media, basically involving the pars tensa, both in the pathogenesis as well as the treatment required to correct the condition. Combined surgery, both through the ear canal and mastoid to eradicate all cholesteatoma with preservation of the pars tensa, posterior external auditory canal, and ear canal skin is the preferred treatment. Physical obliteration of the epitympanum helps to avoid recurrent disease.

Type V: Disease Involving the Middle Ear, Epitympanum, and Mastoid Without Cholesteatoma

Extensive, intractable infectious involvement of the middle ear, epitympanum, and mastoid with perforation of the pars tensa and polypoid hyperplasia is characteristic of this category (Fig 62–1E). It is important to distinguish this condition from that involving cholesteatoma and squamous epithelium within the tympanum, epitympanum, and mastoid. The pathology is basically that of a central perforation of the pars tensa with extensive infection of the mastoid. The condition requires surgical drainage of the mastoid before resolution can be expected and involves the removal of the majority, but not all, of the obstructing granulation tissue; establishment of drainage through the facial recess; and graft of the tympanic membrane without disturbing the edematous mucous membrane around the ossicular chain that is obstructing the attic. Excellent results can be obtained with relatively minimal surgery, although it is for a patient with this type that an inexperienced surgeon might mistakenly perform a radical mastoidectomy.

Type VI: Disease Involving the Middle Ear, Epitympanum, and Mastoid With Cholesteatoma

This category is a combination of types I, II, III, IV, and V. As in type V, otorrhea is generally constant despite all forms of systemic and topical antibiotic treatment. Otoscopic examination usually shows both cholesteatoma and granulation tissue within the middle ear and with extension into the mastoid (Fig 62–1F). Treatment is directed to removal of cholesteatoma, first through a transcanal approach and second by a postauricular approach, working through the facial recess. The tympanic membrane is grafted and drainage is established from the Eustachian tube to the mastoid. Second-stage reconstruction of hearing is usually required.

Discussion

A number of subclassifications could be considered, but do not have the significant implications of these major categories. Before tympanoplasty, great importance was placed on the determination of a marginal perforation because it was that category that often involved invasion of squamous epithelium into the middle ear and would be more troublesome or potentially dangerous. Today, the position of the perforation in the pars tensa has little real signficance other than for the details of surgical repair. The atelectatic ear involves loss of the fibrous layer, which allows the retraction of the pars tensa with the normal development of a 4-cm water vacuum between normal periodic openings of the Eustachian tube. Treatment by myringotomy and insertion of a ventilating tube will allow the thin tympanic membrane to return to its normal position. This is not disease of the Eustachian tube in any way and treatment involves construction of a strong tympanic membrane. The existing two layers must be removed and discarded. The use of this classification in the examination room allows determination of the expected progression of the disease and establishment of the correct medical and surgical treatment.

References

1. Pulec JL, Deguine C. Classification of chronic suppurative otitis media. *Operative Tech Otolaryngol Head Neck Surg.* 1995;6(1):2–4. Copyright 1995 W. B. Saunders. Reprinted with permission.

63

A Surgical System of Management of Chronic Suppurative Otitis Media

The goals of myringoplasty, tympanoplasty, and mastoidectomy in the treatment of chronic suppurative otitis media are:

1. Complete removal of the disease and squamous epithelium from the middle ear and mastoid
2. Preservation of the posterior bony external auditory canal
3. Aeration of the middle ear and in some cases the mastoid
4. Preservation or restoration of useful hearing with complete elimination of an air-bone gap
5. Permanent closure of the tympanic membrane perforation with production of a dry, trouble-free ear

A surgical system of management for the different types of chronic suppurative otitis media has evolved. It is convenient to classify the area and amount of involvement of the ear by disease so that a method of management can be outlined and the patient can be preoperatively apprised of the extent and type of surgery required. Depending on the area and extent of involvement, predetermined surgical procedures can be used, either alone or together, as building blocks that can be called on when needed. A useful system of surgical units includes (1) myringoplasty, (2) tympanoplasty with intact tympanic membrane, (3) myringoplasty combined with tympanoplasty, (4) transcanal removal of attic cholesteatoma and mastoidectomy with removal of cholesteatoma, (5) myringoplasty with removal of obstructing granulation tissue from the tympanum and mastoidectomy to estabish drainage through the facial recess, and (6) myringoplasty in combination with tympanoplasty and mastoidectomy for the removal of an extensive cholesteatoma. In addition, special techniques are required for the management of complications. By using these individual surgical procedures, alone or together, gratify-

ing results can be obtained with preservation of the external auditory canal, removal of cholesteatoma, and effective reconstruction of hearing.

The Roman numeral of the type of tympanoplasty required is the same as the Roman numeral of the type of chronic suppurative otitis media in our classification. The six types of tympanoplasty are as follows:

Type I: Myringoplasty

Type II: Transcanal tympanoplasty with intact tympanic membrane

Type III: Myringoplasty and tympanoplasty combined

Type IV: Transcanal removal of attic cholesteatoma and mastoidectomy

Type V: Myringoplasty, tympanoplasty, and mastoidectomy with drainage through the facial recess

Type VI: Myringoplasty, tympanoplasty, and mastoidectomy with removal of cholesteatoma

For a detailed description of the surgical techniques, the reader is referred to the bibliography.

Bibliography

1. Pulec JL, guest ed. Surgery for chronic suppurative otitis media. *Operative Tech Otolaryngol Head Neck Surg.* 1995;6(1).
2. Pulec JL. A surgical system of management of chronic suppurative otitis media. *Operative Tech Otolaryngol Head Neck Surg.* 1995;6(1):5–16.
3. Pulec JL. Sinus tympani: surgical approach for the removal of cholesteatoma. *Ear Nose Throat J.* 1996; 75(2):77–88.
4. Pulec JL. Labyrinthine fistula from cholesteatoma: surgical management. *Ear Nose Throat J.* 1996;75(3): 143–148.

64

A Basic Principle of Tympanoplasty Surgery: Anterior Perforation of the Pars Tensa With and Without Obstructed View

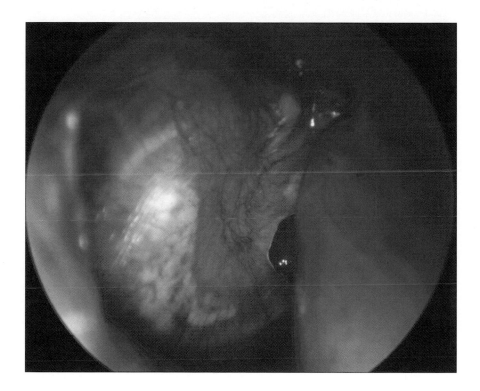

Fig 64–1

Obstructed View

With rare exceptions a clear view of the entire operative site including the entire annulus is essential to obtain reliable success in tympanoplasty. The otoscopic view in Figure 64–1 is of a right ear demonstrating a dry perforation of the anterior inferior quadrant of the pars tensa. From the right side of the photograph a large anterior bony canal wall bulge obliterates the view of the perforation and the anterior annulus. It is absolutely necessary to elevate the skin from the anterior canal wall and remove the obstructing bone until the entire anterior annulus can be seen. Use of the canal skin would be the most desirable method of repair.

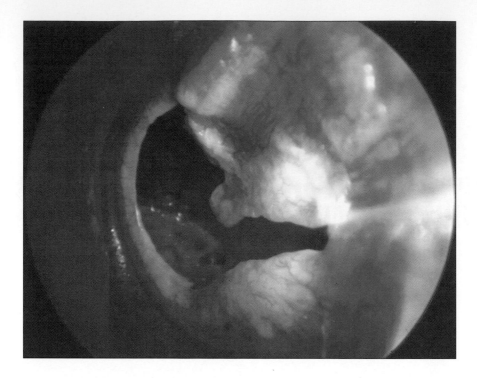

Fig 64–2

Unobstructed View

The otoscopic view in Figure 64–2 is of a left ear with a large anterior perforation of the pars tensa. The entire anterior annulus can be seen and it is not necessary to remove bone from the anterior canal wall to obtain a good view. The anterior canal wall bulge obstructs the view of the anterior sulcus in 30% of all ears.

Atlas of Otoscopy

65

Classification of Chronic Suppurative Otitis Media: Type I

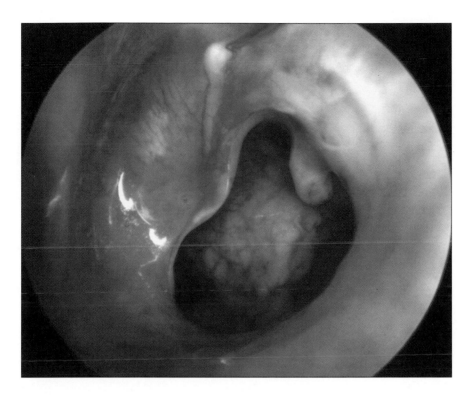

Fig 65–1

The authors proposed a classification of chronic suppurative otitis media, which was published in *Operative Techniques in Otolaryngology—Head and Neck Surgery* (1995;6[1]:2–4). We feel that the classification is a useful tool for the clinician as he or she examines patients in the office. One of six distinct categories can be identified by the otoscopic examination. These categories include:

Type I: Perforation of the tympanic membrane alone without evidence of other disease.

Type II: Conductive hearing loss with intact tympanic membrane.

Type III: Tympanic membrane perforation with disease confined to the middle ear and epitympanum.

Type IV: Attic cholesteatoma.

Type V: Disease involving the middle ear, epitympanum, and mastoid without cholesteatoma.

Type VI: Disease involving the middle ear, epitympanum, and mastoid with cholesteatoma.

The classification of the disease corresponds to a similar classification of the surgical procedure required. This system in valuable to the surgeon who is trained to do transcanal procedures, preservation of the intact posterior external auditory canal in all cases, and especially the routine total removal of all cholesteatoma basement membrane. This chapter and the next five describe this classification. Type I chronic suppurative chronic otitis media involves only perforation of the pars tensa without other disease. Treatment required is a type I tympanoplasty not unlike that described by Professor Horst Wulstein.

66

Classification of Chronic Suppurative Otitis Media: Type II

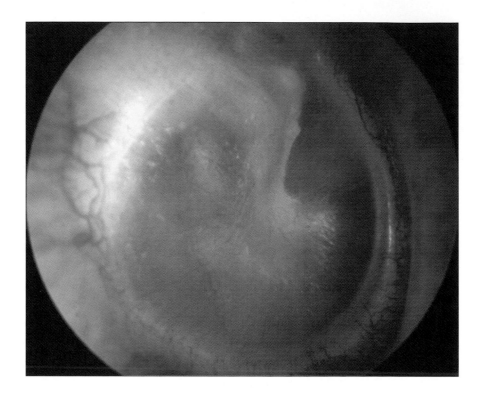

Fig 66–1

This is the second in a series of six chapters describing a classification of chronic suppurative otitis media proposed by the authors, which was published in *Operative Techniques in Otolaryngology — Head and Neck Surgery* (1995;6[1]:2–4).

Type II: Conductive Hearing Loss With Intact Tympanic Membrane

The otoscopic examination shows a right ear that appears completely normal. There is no visible evidence of a healed perforation or tympanosclerosis, although the ear has a conductive hearing loss due to the effects of previous chronic otitis media. The diagnosis is suspected from the history and, in some cases, the use of impedance audiometry. The differential diagnosis may include conductive hearing loss caused by fixation of the ossicular chain by a congenital fixation of bone, Paget's disease, by tympanosclerosis involving the ossicular chain, fracture or dislocation of the ossicular chain from trauma or dissolution of part of the ossicular chain from infection or immunologic effects. Otosclerosis must be considered. Treatment is directed to restoration of the hearing. Ossicular reconstruction and middle-ear work can be performed through a tympano-meatal flap similar to that required for a stapedectomy.

67

Classification of Chronic Suppurative Otitis Media: Type III

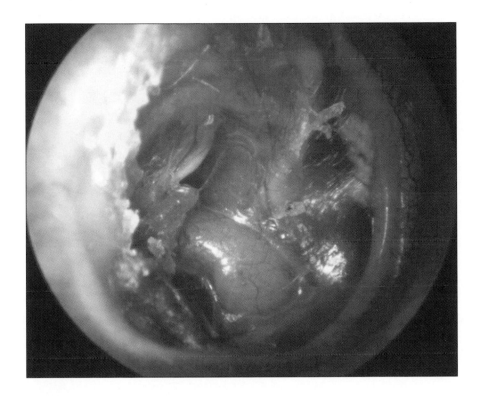

Fig 67–1

This is the third in a series of six chapters describing the classification of chronic suppurative otitis media proposed by the authors and published in *Operative Techniques in Otolaryngology—Head and Neck Surgery* (1995;6[1]:2–4).

Type III: Tympanic Membrane Perforation With Disease Confined to the Middle Ear and Epitympanum

This category involves a combination of type I and type II with the addition of the possibility of cholesteatoma and squamous epithelium involving the tympanic cavity. There may be a central perfo-ration with squamous epithelium extending onto the medial surface of the pars tensa or the squamous epithelium may extend over the promontory and seal off the tubotympanum. This category includes forms of adhesive otitis media in which the tympanic membrane is retracted and adherent to the promontory. The goal of treatment is not only to restore hearing but also to eliminate infection and to reconstruct the tympanic membrane. The surgical procedure of choice is performed entirely through a speculum through the external auditory canal and often requires the placement of Silastic film in the tympanum to prevent adhesions. Reconstruction is done at a second stage.

68

Classification of Chronic Suppurative Otitis Media: Type IV

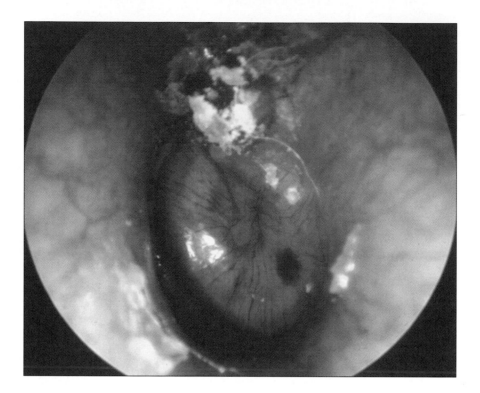

Fig 68–1

This is the fourth in the series of six chapters describing classification of chronic suppurative otitis media proposed by the authors, which was published in *Operative Techniques in Otolaryngology— Head and Neck Surgery* (1995;6[1]:2–4).

Type IV: Attic Cholesteatoma

Attic cholesteatoma develops as an expanding herniation of the pars flaccida into the epitympanum, mastoid, and middle ear. Except in the most advanced cases, the pars tensa is uninvolved. This type of cholesteatoma usually remains dry and free of drainage unless the cholesteatomatous debris

becomes wet and infected. Its development is insidious, with progressive, conductive hearing loss and eventually the development of a labyrinthine fistula or facial paralysis. The condition is significantly different from chronic suppurative otitis media, basically involving the pars tensa, both in the pathogenesis as well as the treatment required to correct the condition. Combined surgery, through both the ear canal and mastoid, to eradicate all cholesteatoma with preservation of the pars tensa, posterior external bony canal, and ear canal skin is the preferred treatment. Physical obliteration of the epitympanum helps to avoid recurrent disease.

69

Classification Of Chronic Suppurative Otitis Media: Type V

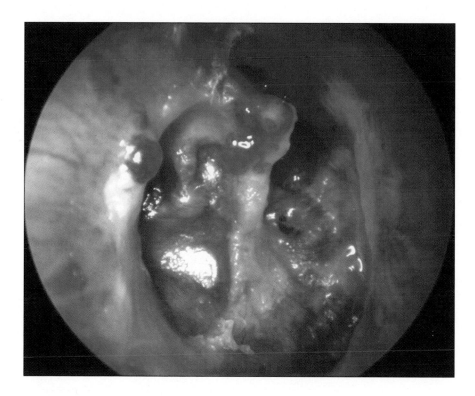

Fig 69–1

This is the fifth in the series of six chapters describing the classification of chronic suppurative otitis media proposed by the authors and published in *Operative Techniques in Otolaryngology—Head and Neck Surgery* (1995;6[1]:2–4).

Type V: Disease Involving the Middle Ear, Epitympanum, and Mastoid Without Cholesteatoma

Extensive intractable infectious involvement of the middle ear, epitympanum, and mastoid, with perforation of the pars tensa and polypoid hyperplasia is characteristic of this category. It is important to distinguish this condition from that involving cholesteatoma and squamous epithelium within the tympanum, epitympanum, and mastoid. The pathology is basically that of a central perforation of the pars tensa with extensive infection of the mastoid. The condition requires surgical drainage of the mastoid before resolution can be expected, and involves the removal of the majority, but not all, of the obstructing granulation tissue, establishment of drainage through the facial recess, and grafting of the tympanic membrane without disturbing the edematous mucous membrane around the ossicular chain that is obstructing the attic. Excellent results can be obtained with relatively minimal surgery, although it is for a patient with this type of chronic suppurative otitis media that an inexperienced surgeon might mistakenly perform a radical mastoidectomy.

Classification of Chronic Suppurative Otitis Media: Type VI

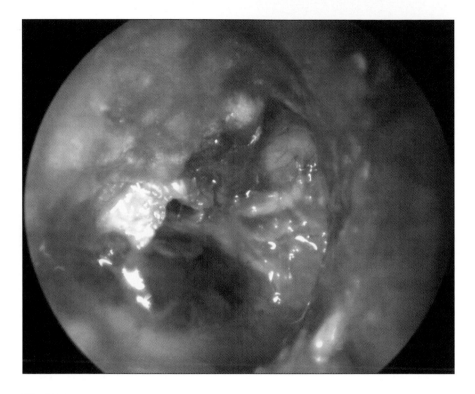

Fig 70–1

This is the sixth and final chapter in the series of six chapters describing classification of chronic suppurative otitis media proposed by the authors, which was published in *Operative Techniques in Otolaryngology—Head and Neck Surgery* (1995;6[1]: 2–4).

Type VI: Disease Involving the Middle Ear

This category is a combination of types I, II, III, IV, and V. As in Type V, otorrhea is generally constant despite all forms of systemic and topical antibiotic treatment. Otoscopic examination usually shows both cholesteatoma and granulation tissue within the middle ear and with extension into the mastoid. Treatment is directed to removal of cholesteatoma, first through a transcanal approach and second by a postauricular approach, working through the facial recess. The tympanic membrane is grafted and drainage is established from the mastoid to the Eustachian tube. Second-stage reconstruction of hearing is usually required.

71

Dry Central Tympanic Membrane Perforation

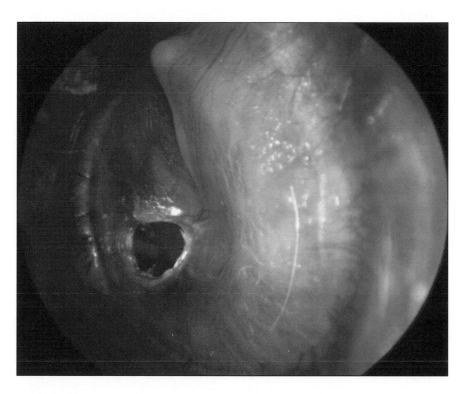

Fig 71–1

The dry central perforation of the tympanic membrane secondary to trauma or infection may be entirely asymptomatic. Small perforations of the tympanic membrane seldom produce detectable hearing loss. They may be found incidentally during routine examination or their presence may be suspected when the patient gives a history of repeated episodes of otorrhea after water enters the ear followed by long periods without symptoms. The otoscopic view reveals a left tympanic membrane with a completely normal pars tensa with the exception of a 2-mm dry perforation immediately anterior and inferior to the umbo. The medial wall of the tympanum can be seen through the perforation just at the edge of the tubotympanum. There is no evidence of purulent, mucoid, or serous drainage. There is no blood clot and no inflammation. A thin, almost white rim of proliferating mucous membrane and squamous epithelium represents an unsuccessful attempt at spontaneous healing. A yellow thickened mass at the superior edge of the perforation appears like a retracted and folded portion of the fibrous layer and suggests that the perforation might have been traumatic in origin. Ninety percent of all traumatic pars tensa perforations heal spontaneously within 4 weeks. The 10% of traumatic perforations that fail to heal after 4 weeks and other dry central perforations are surgically repaired on an elective basis. Extremely small perforations may be treated by surgically excising a ½-mm ring of the circumference of the perforation and placing a paper patch, for example, a disc of stationery, on the freshly bleeding perforation. Should that technique be unsuccessful, an underlay or overlay myringoplasty graft technique will usually result in successful permanent closure of the perforation.

72

Microperforation of the Pars Tensa Due to a Hair

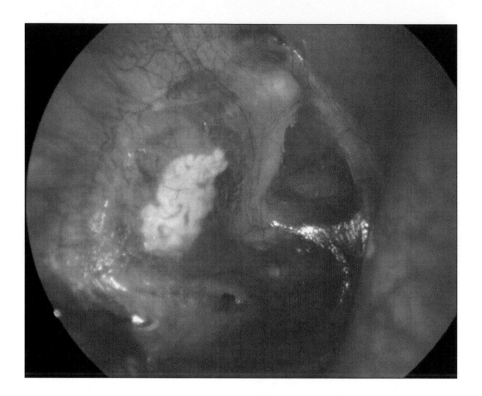

Fig 72–1

The otoscopic view is that of a right ear demonstrating a small pinpoint perforation of the pars tensa that occurred due to a hair that grew against the tympanic membrane. In addition, there is a patch of white tympanosclerosis occupying the posterior, superior quadrant of the pars tensa. The pars tensa appears otherwise intact and normal. Halfway between the umbo and the annulus in line with the handle of the malleus, a pinpoint perforation is seen through the pars tensa. It is dry and there is no evidence of infection. A dark-colored hair growing from the anterior, external auditory canal wall is

seen extending through the perforation of the pars tensa. There is no infection or drainage. Hair growing against the tympanic membrane can occasionally (usually once every 4 or 5 years) produce an annoying symptom of tinnitus. Simple removal of the hair will solve the problem until the hair again grows against the tympanic membrane. Rarely, the hair will produce a perforation. In such a situation the hair must be removed, and a minor repair of the perforation made, usually by excising the edges of the perforation under a local anesthetic in the office and covering it with a patch is satisfactory treatment.

Atlas of Otoscopy

73

Slag Burn Tympanic Membrane Perforation

The otoscopic view demonstrates a small anterior perforation of the par tensa at low- (Figure 73–1) and high-power (Figure 73–2) magnification. There is no otorrhea or local inflammation and, at first glance, it would appear to respond successfully to any type of myringoplasty. In fact, when one knows the history—the perforation was caused by a burn from a hot piece of metal —these cases can be difficult to repair and often give disappointing results. The injury is most commonly caused when a molten piece of metal enters the ear when a workman is using an arc welder or an acetylene torch, and less commonly, from molten solder or when a grinder is being used. The exact reason that this lesion is prone to surgical failure when normal techniques are used is not entirely clear. The high-magnification otoscopic view, however, demonstrates an area of injury beyond that of the perforation itself. Surgical success can be expected if the surgeon is aware of the problem and takes special care with technique. It is necessary to resect all of the injured tissue surrounding the perforation and to use a graft material such as perichondrium or substantial fascia. The final perforation to be grafted is often much larger than that which is originally seen in the examination room. A lateral technique that includes desquamation of the entire pars tensa and placement of the graft lateral to the fibrous layer seems to give the best results.

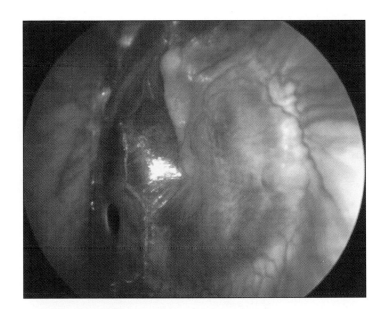

Fig 73–1

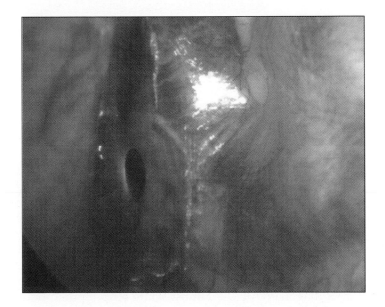

Fig 73–2

74

Dry Central Total Tympanic Membrane Perforation

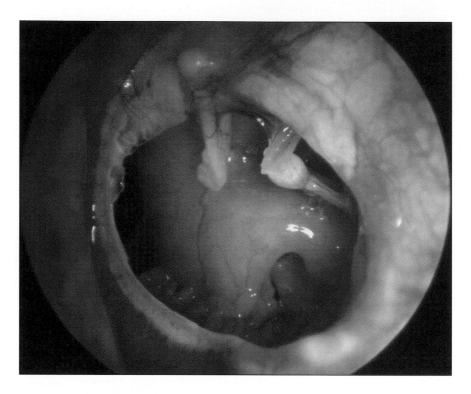

Fig 74–1

The otoscopic view shown above is that of a left dry central perforation involving almost all of the pars tensa. Only the fibrous annulus and a very small remnant of the pars tensa at the anterior superior area remain. The naked handle of the malleus devoid of any pars tensa protrudes into the center of the perforation. The short process of the malleus protrudes up from the slightly erythematous pars flaccida at the superior edge of the photograph with the handle of the malleus extending inferiorly to end in a slightly larger whitish mass that is the umbo. This looks something like the pendulum of a clock. At the posterior superior edge of the perforation, a diagonally placed almost white strip represents the chorda tympani passing from the area of the short process of the malleus to its canal in the posterior bony canal wall. Anterior and inferior to

this can be seen part of the long process of the incus, the lenticular process of the incus, the incudostapedial joint, and the stapedius tendon as it passes from the pyramid to the stapes. Medial to the incus is a darkened depression, which represents the oval window. Inferior to the stapes can be seen the round window niche and in its uppermost area the glistening round window membrane. Through the perforation, the glistening mucous membrane over the whitish bone of the promontory is visible. Capillaries cross the promontory in an inferior to superior direction. The dark area seen through the anterior part of the perforation is the tubotympanum. Perforations of this size often produce a 30–50 dB HL conductive hearing loss. Recurrent infections follow the installation of water into the middle ear or occur during a head cold. Treatment involves the elective and desirable performance of myringoplasty. No Silastic film is required if care is taken to avoid abrasion of the normal mucous membrane of the promontory. Almost any accepted graft material can be used with success, although repair with a homograft tympanic membrane covered with canal skin can successfully restore both normal appearance and hearing.

75

Dry Central Tympanic Membrane Perforation And Tympanosclerosis

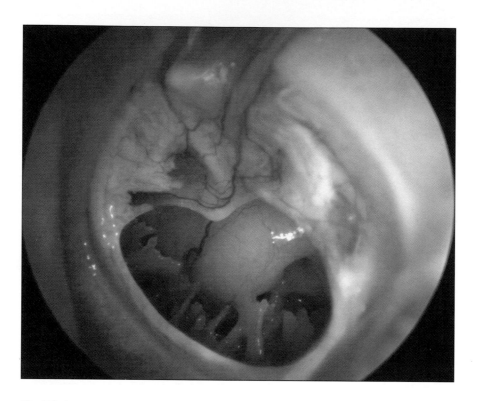

Fig 75–1

This is an otoscopic view of a left ear with a 60% dry central perforation of the pars tensa and patches of tympanosclerosis involving the tympanic membrane remnant. There is no evidence of infection, cholesteatoma, or involvement of the tympanum. The perforation is heart-shaped with a superior notch in the area of the umbo. The pars flaccida is normal and there is an area of normal pars tensa both anterior and posterior to the malleus. Several small bright-red capillaries can be seen extending from the superior bony canal wall along the long process of the malleus. Tympanosclerosis can be seen as patches of thickened white mass that replace the fibrous annulus. Through the perforation the normal structures of the medial wall of the tympanum are observed. The normal irregular bone formation of the hypotympanum changes to the smooth glistening surface of the promontory over which courses

a bright red capillary in the area of the tympanic nerve. A round window niche is seen posterior and inferior to the umbo. A light reflex is immediately superior to the round window. Although one cannot tell with certainty, this ear most likely has no fixation. The tympanosclerosis is most likely confined to the tympanic membrane remnant and is primarily cosmetic. Tympanosclerosis is the result of an immune response in the body's healing process similar to the ingrowth of squamous epithelium. Treatment is elective and should be conservative. Successful perforation closure is expected and good hearing depends on the surgeon's technique. Several methods can be used without removing the drum remnant, including underlay fascia or overlay canal skin and periosteum techniques. Complete replacement of the pars tensa using a homograft tympanic membrane and canal skin can yield excellent results.

76

Cholesteatoma With Intact Tympanic Membrane

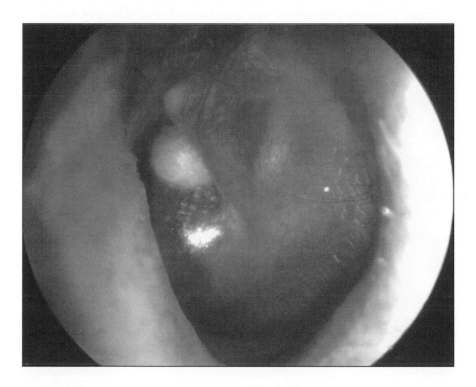

Fig 76–1

This otoscopic view of a left ear shows a completely normal tympanic membrane. The malleus is vertical and the short process is seen at its upper edge as a cream-colored protrusion. The pars tensa is intact, and there is a good light reflex at the center of the photograph. The promontory is barely seen through the center of the pars tensa. The incus appears at the right upper edge of the tympanic membrane. The prominent feature is a spherical cream-colored mass seen through the translucent pars tensa anterior to the malleus. This represents cholesteatoma within the middle ear. Once these were thought to be congenital rests of epithelium, but it has now been shown that they are acquired and there is a healed, grossly invisible fistula to account for the entrance of squamous epithelium into the tympanum. The true congenital cholesteatoma normally involves the cerebellopontine angle or temporal bone, and clearly extends from the temporal bone into the middle ear. Treatment is to surgically excise the cholesteatoma completely. If attachment to the pars tensa is identified the fistulous tract must be excised and the area grafted.

77

Cholesteatoma With Intact Tympanic Membrane

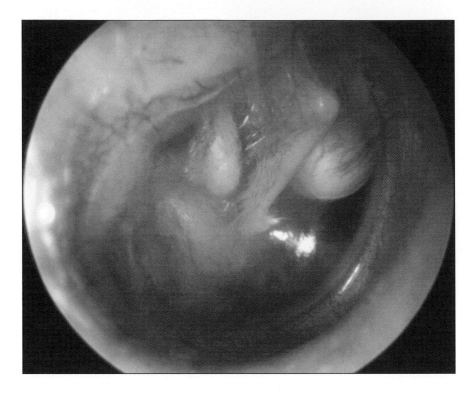

Fig 77–1

The otoscopic view is that of a right ear of a 5-year-old boy. The external auditory canal, tympanic membrane, malleus, incus, and middle ear are normal with the exception of a solitary spherical, 3-mm cream-colored mass in the tympanum visible through the anterior superior quadrant of the pars tensa. There is no visible perforation of the pars tensa. The tympanum contains no fluid or infection. Hearing is normal. Total removal of the cholesteatoma with excision of a small part of the overlying pars tensa that might contain a micro-fistula and subsequent grafting is indicated. The procedure can be performed through the external canal.

78

Footplate Otosclerosis and Tympanic Membrane Perforation

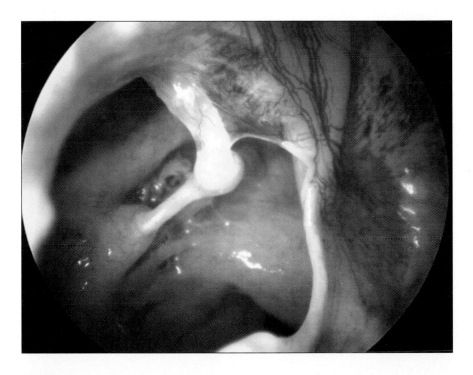

Fig 78–1

The otoscopic view is that of a right ear with a dry perforation involving the posterior 50% of the pars tensa, allowing the observer an unusual opportunity to see the otosclerosis fixing the anterior part of the stapes footplate. The ear is dry and the anterior half of the pars tensa is intact. Through the posterior perforation, which extends from the handle of the malleus to the posterior annular rim, can be seen the cream-colored promontory of the tympanum. At the inferior edge of the perforation, the round window niche is visible. Posterior and superior to the round window niche is the infrapyramidal recess, the pyramid and stapedius tendon, and the oval window and the stapes. Superior to the oval window niche is the fallopian canal. The lenticular process of the incus is intact but thinned and partially eroded. A thin film of mucous membrane extends from the incus to the malleus superior to the incudostapedial joint. Inferior to this filamentous membrane and superior to the capitulum of the stapes can be seen the anterior crus of the stapes and the anterior edge of the oval window, which are involved with a whitish-red otosclerotic focus. Clinical confirmation of the presence of otosclerosis was made by the presence of fixation of the stapes in the opposite ear in the absence of a perforation in the tympanic membrane. The left ear had a conductive hearing loss that was completely eliminated by successful stapedectomy. Myringoplasty was performed on the right ear, and after a reasonable period of healing, right stapedectomy was performed. The advent of widespread vaccination for rubella and its eradication will no doubt lead to the elimination of clinical otosclerosis.

79

Dry Central Tympanic Membrane Perforation With Tympanosclerosis

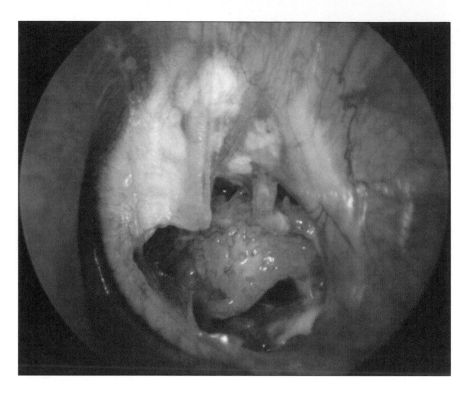

Fig 79–1

The otoscopic photograph is of the left ear and represents two pathologic changes of otitis media. The ear is dry with no evidence of infection. A 60% dry central perforation of the pars tensa exposes the mucous membrane of the promontory. Several patches of white opaque thickened tympanosclerosis can be seen in the drum remnant. A large patch of tympanosclerosis almost completely replaces the remnant anterior to the malleus. Several smaller patches are seen around the short process of the malleus. Posterior to the malleus, the chorda tympani is seen at the superior part of the photograph. The drum remnant posterior to the malleus is two-layered and has an adhesion to the long process of the incus. This two-layered tympanic membrane has several patches of tympanosclerosis replacing the fibrous layer. The long process of the incus is clearly seen and is attached to the capitulum of the stapes in a normal fashion. At the bottom of the photograph, the darkened round window niche is visible. From this view, it is impossible to determine whether there is fixation of the ossicular chain. If there is no fixation, transcanal myringoplasty using canal skin or other graft material can be performed with the tympanosclerotic plaques left in place. Should fixation be present, the tympanum is removed and tympanoplasty through the transcanal approach using a homograft tympanic membrane and canal skin is the treatment of choice.

80

Extensive Tympanosclerosis and Short Incus

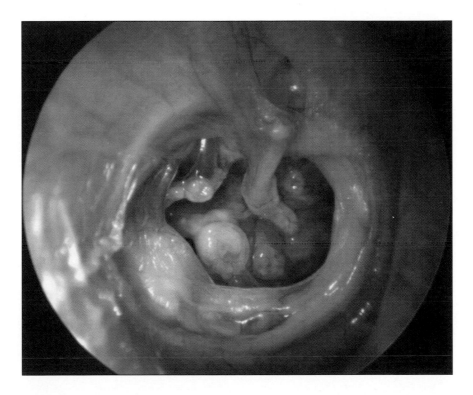

Fig 80–1

The otoscopic view is that of a right ear with chronic otitis media. There is a large central perforation of the pars tensa, a short incus, and extensive, cream-colored tympanosclerosis involving the tympanic membrane remnant, the malleus, the stapes, and the promontory of the tympanum. Tympanosclerosis involves the anterior suspensory ligament of the malleus and a mucous membrane adhesion from the umbo to the promontory. Tympanosclerosis also involves the stapedius tendon and a mucosal fold extending from the capitulum of the stapes to the cochleariform process. Through the perforation in the pars tensa can be seen mounds of cream-colored tympanosclerosis covered with mucous membrane. A large mass is visible anterior to the round window niche. There is no evidence of cho-

lesteatoma within the tympanum and no infection. This ear would likely benefit from a two-stage tympanoplasty performed under a local anesthetic through the external auditory canal. The first procedure would involve removal of the tympanosclerosis of the tympanic membrane remnant and the masses fixing the malleus and the stapes. This would most likely involve removal of the head of the malleus, the stapes tendon, and the mucosal folds between these ossicles and the tympanum. The tympanic membrane would be grafted. Thin Silastic film would be used to prevent adhesions between the graft and the promontory. A second-stage procedure would involve use of a prosthesis between the mobile capitulum of the stapes and the malleus or tympanic membrane graft.

81

Extensive Tympanosclerosis
With Fixed Malleus

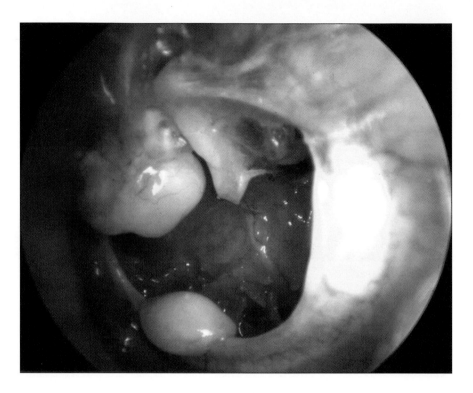

Fig 81–1

The otoscopic view is that of a right ear demonstrating extensive tympanosclerosis of the tympanic membrane only. Through a large perforation in the pars tensa, the normal mucous membrane-covered promontory of the tympanum and the normal stapes and incus can be seen. The pars flaccida appears normal. There are three masses of tympanosclerosis involving the pars tensa. The plaque within the tympanic membrane remnant is seen at the posterior edge of the remnant. A spherical mass involves the inferior edge of the perforation. A larger spherical mass extends from the anterior to the superior edge of the tympanic membrane perforation and involves the anterior suspensory ligament of the malleus, fixing the malleus. A one-stage tympanoplasty performed under a local anesthetic through a speculum in the external auditory canal would likely offer success. All three areas of tympanosclerosis would be removed in this case and a tympanic membrane graft would be used. It is important to obtain approximately 2 mm of space between the anterior bony annulus and the mobilized malleus to prevent refixation in that area. No Silastic film is required.

82

Tympanic Membrane Perforation and Tympanosclerosis With Ossicular Fixation

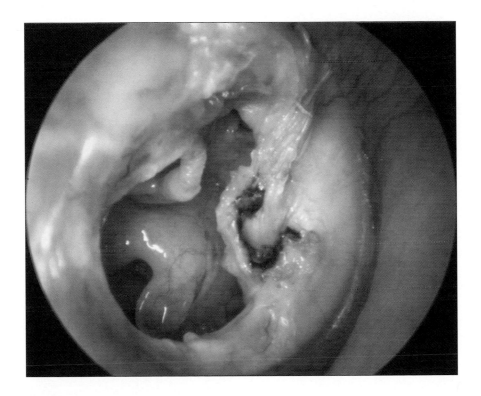

Fig 82–1

The otoscopic photograph of the right ear represents the effects of otitis media. There is a dry, 50% posterior perforation of the pars tensa, with extensive involvement by tympanosclerosis of the anterior drum remnant. Squamous epithelium can be seen at the edge of the anterior part of the perforation and within the middle ear. The fibrous layer of the tympanic membrane is extensively involved with a thick, white mass of tympanosclerosis that fixes the malleus. The amount of extension of squamous epithelium medial to the tympanic membrane remnant can be minimal or extensive. The chorda tympani is seen at the posterior superior edge of the perforation. The lenticular process of the incus is slightly eroded but intact and in contact with a normal stapes. At the inferior edge of the perforation, the round window membrane can be seen as a dark oval. The tympanic nerve and the artery with it cross the promontory in a vertical direction from the hypotympanum to the cochleariform process. The tendon of the tensor tympani muscle can be seen at the superior edge of the perforation. Squamous epithelium commonly extends over a part of the medial side of the tympanic membrane when tympanosclerosis is present. Treatment involves tympanoplasty through a speculum, usually under a local anesthetic. The tympanic membrane remnant, including the tympanosclerosis, is completely removed, along with all squamous epithelium basement membrane within the tympanum. Reconstruction is best accomplished with a homograft tympanic membrane and canal skin. Ossicular fixation, if it persists, is handled by second-stage tympanoplasty.

83

Short Incus and Posterior Perforation Healed With a Retracted Neomembrane

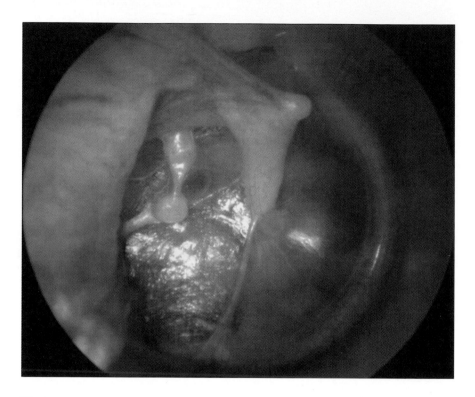

Fig 83–1

The otoscopic photograph is of a right ear and represents the effects of otitis media. There is no evidence of active infection, serous fluid, or otorrhea. The pars flaccida is intact and appears normal. The malleus appears as a pale cream-colored bone extending from the superior edge of the annular ring to the center of the photograph where the round umbo covered by pars flaccida is seen. The short process of the malleus protrudes laterally and anteriorly into the external auditory canal. A line, representing a fold in the tympanic membrane and the edge of a healed perforation, extends in line with and inferior to the manubrium of the malleus to the inferior edge of the annulus. Anterior to this line the intact completely normal pars flaccida appears translucent. In the anterior superior quadrant the dark area represents the tubotympanum.

At the inferior edge the dark area is the hypotympanum. The posterior half of the pars tensa is replaced by a thin two-layered neomembrane. This thin membrane is intact, but does not have the strength to withstand the vacuum of 4 cm of water that normally develops between periodic opening of the Eustachian tube. The membrane is retracted and adherent to the chorda tympani nerve which passes medial to the neck of the malleus and lateral to the long process of the incus near the superior edge of the tympanum. The lentricular process of the incus is eroded leaving a ¼-mm strand of fibrous tissue connecting the remnant of the long process of the incus to a remnant of the ventricular process of the surface of the capitulum of the stapes. Immediately inferior to this strand is the stapes lying almost perpendicular to the long process of the incus and malleus. The stapedius tendon is a white structure seen just lateral to the posterior crus of the stapes between the capitulum of the stapes and the pyramid. The pyramid cannot be seen because the posterior canal wall obstructs our view of it. Inferior to the stapes the neomembrane is adherent to the promontory just superior to the darkened round window niche. Superior to the stapes and immediately medial to the remnant of the short incus lies on the cream-colored fallopian canal. Treatment involves tympanoplasty by reconstruction of a strong tympanic membrane and placement of an ossicle or prosthesis between the mobile malleus or tympanic membrane graft. If hearing is normal because of the myringostapedopexy and the patient is otherwise symptom free, no treatment is required.

84

Short Incus With Intact Tympanic Membrane

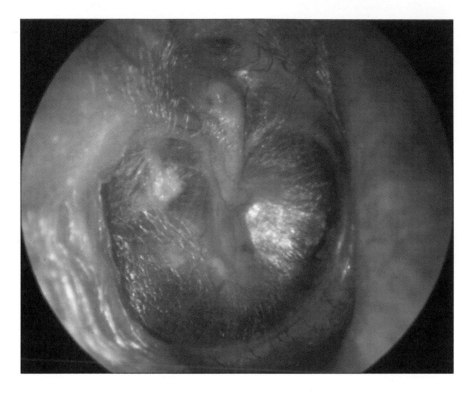

Fig 84–1

The otoscopic photograph is of the right ear and represents the effects of otitis media. There is no evidence of active infection, serous fluid, or otorrhea. The malleus is normal. The pars tensa is a thin two-layered flaccid membrane, which appears slightly retracted in its entire area. The retraction medial to and slightly posterior to the posterior bony annulus prevents a portion of the membrane from being seen. Especially notable is the white 1-mm spot in the posterior-superior quadrant that is the lenticular process of the incus attached to the capitulum of the stapes. The thin tympanic membrane seems to be lying against the lenticular process or might be adherent to it. The incus is eroded and short so that it does not quite connect with the lenticular process. The remnant of the long process can be seen posterior and superior to the lenticular process and the capitulum of the stapes. Should hearing be normal and the patient be free of other symptoms, no treatment is required. A conductive hearing loss is treated by two stages of surgery, both done by a transcanal approach through a speculum. The first procedure involves using a homograft tympanic membrane to repair the pars tensa. After 4 months a sculptured bone strut is placed between the capitulum and the manubrium of the malleus or tympanic membrane.

85

Atelectasis and Chronic Suppurative Otitis Media

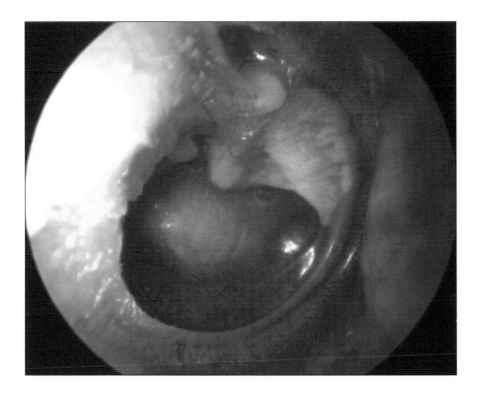

Fig 85–1

The otoscopic view shows a left ear that has three separate conditions in association with chronic suppurative otitis media. It represents Type III chronic otitis media as previously described by the authors.[1] There is atelectasis of the thin two-layered neomembrane, which has the appearance of a 70% perforation of the pars tensa. Serous fluid is seen through the translucent tympanic membrane. The membrane is draped over and adherent to the promontory. The lenticular process of the incus can be seen at the superior edge of the perforation. The malleus is retracted and appears to be shortened. There is a retraction of the pars flaccida into the epitympanum with the appearance of serous fluid behind the retracted membrane. The anterior superior quarter of the pars tensa is involved in tympanosclerosis. Surgical treatment of this type of ear pathology requires a type III myringoplasty and tympano-plasty, combined as previously described by Pulec.[2] A few weeks before the surgery is performed, myringotomy with insertion of a ventilating button is accomplished with the intent to restore the atelectatic portion of the tympanic membrane to its normal position, aerate the middle ear, and simplify the surgery by eliminating the need for hazardous dissection of squamous epithelium from the medial wall of the ear and ossicular chain. At the time of surgery, the tympanosclerosis that is likely fixing the malleus must be removed and a strong, new pars tensa must be constructed. This type of ear frequently needs long-term ventilation with a tympanostomy tube to maintain aeration of the middle ear and good hearing. A Wright Eustachian tube prosthesis sometimes provides long-term relief from recurrent serous otitis media.

References

1. Pulec J, Deguine C. Classification of suppurative otitis media. *Operative Tech Otolaryngol Head Neck Surg.* 1995;6(1):2–4.

2. Pulec J. A surgical system of management of chronic suppurative otitis media. *Operative Tech Otolaryngol Head Neck Surg.* 1995;6(1):5-16.

86

Dry Central Perforation With Squamous Epithelium in the Tympanum

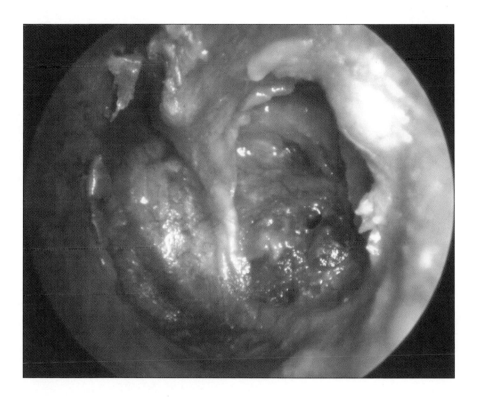

Fig 86–1

Cases of chronic otitis media that involve ingrowth of squamous epithelium through a perforation to cover the surfaces of the tympanum challenge the skill of the well-trained otologic surgeon. Every cell of the basement membrane of the squamous epithelium that has grown into the middle ear must be removed and the raw surface must be covered with Silastic film so that new mucous membrane can grow back and the ear can again be aerated. This is an otoscopic view of a left ear with type III chronic otitis media, as previously described by the authors.[1] There is a 50% posterior perforation of the pars tensa. The anterior drum remnant is involved with tympanosclerosis and it is very likely that squamous epithelium has covered much of the medial surface of the remaining tympanic membrane. The malleus is present but there is no

evidence of the incus or stapes crura. The fallopian canal can be seen through the upper portion of the perforation. The oval window is immediately below the fallopian canal. The entire medial surface of the tympanic membrane is covered with squamous epithelium and it appears that the squamous epithelium extends around the edges of the perforation. Although the majority of cases with this appearance can be satisfactorily treated by a local anesthetic by working through a speculum through the external auditory canal, the surgeon and the patient must be aware that squamous epithelium sometimes extends into the epitympanum and mastoid and that a postauricular incision and an intact external auditory canal wall mastoidectomy might be required. Silastic film is placed in the middle ear to prevent adhesions and to allow regrowth of mucous membrane over the surfaces of the tympanum. The pars tensa and pars flaccida are grafted. Reconstruction of hearing with the placement of a prosthesis between the mobile footplate and the tympanic membrane graft is performed when healing is complete after 4 months.

Reference

1. Pulec J, Deguine C. Classification of chronic suppurative otitis media. *Operative Tech Otolaryngol Head Neck Surg.* 1995;6(1):2–4.

87

Tympanic Membrane Perforation With Squamous Epithelium Within the Tympanum

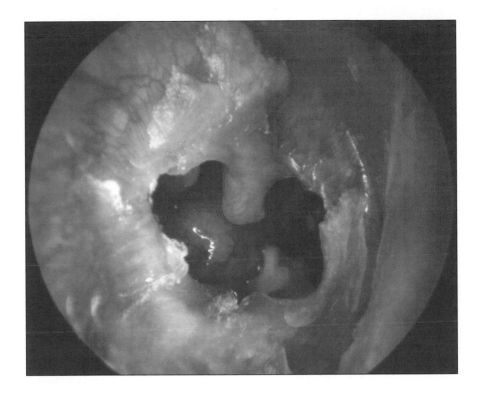

Fig 87–1

The otoscopic photograph is of the right ear and represents progressive otitis media. The remnant of the tympanic membrane is slightly erythematous. A 60% central perforation allows a view of the glistening and slightly edematous mucous membrane on the promontory. A dry yellow crust of intermittent otorrhea is seen on the drum remnant, both superiorly and inferiorly. Squamous epithelium can be seen in the anterior hypotympanum lying on the promontory. At the posterior superior edge of the perforation, the lenticular process of the incus covered with edematous mucosa is seen. Treatment is directed to the creation of a dry ear by the use of systemic antibiotics and topical aqueous ear drops containing steroids and antibiotics for 1 or 2 weeks. Transcanal tympanoplasty is then performed with removal of the squamous epithelium from the tympanum. A disk of Silastic film is placed in the middle ear to prevent adhesions and the tympanic membrane is grafted. A homograft tympanic membrane and canal skin is ideal for reconstruction.

88

Tympanosclerosis With Squamous Epithelium in the Tympanum

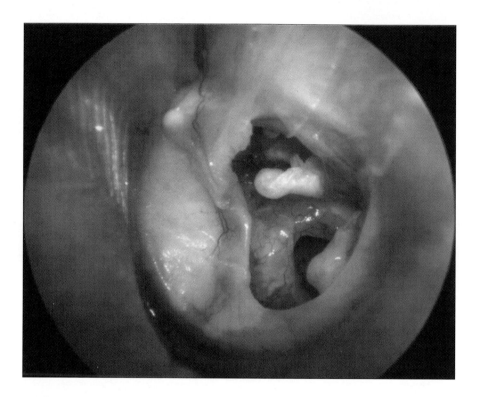

Fig 88–1

The otoscopic view is that of a left ear with a 50% posterior perforation of the pars tensa. The anterior intact drum remnant is involved extensively with tympanosclerosis, the cream-colored thickening of the fibrous layer. The handle of the malleus is seen with the white, short process. Although the mucous membrane of the promontory appears healthy, there are two areas of potential danger. One involves squamous epithelium clearly extending into the tympanum on the undersurface of the pars tensa, especially evident immediately posterior to the long process of the malleus. The roughened area is squamous epithelium extending around the edge of the perforation. It is not possible to tell unless one were to use a telescope to determine how far anteriorly this cholesteatoma extends. The second area of trouble is that of the stapedius tendon and capitulum of the stapes, which is covered with squamous epithelium. This ear requires surgery that involves tympanoplasty under a local anesthetic done through a speculum through the external auditory canal. The entire pars tensa remnant must be removed along with squamous epithelium medial to it. The squamous epithelium involving the stapedius tendon and capitulum must also be removed. It appears that the crura of the stapes and the long process of the incus are missing. An attempt would be made to mobilize the handle of the malleus. A two-stage procedure utilizing Silastic film to prevent adhesions is required. At the second-stage procedure the ossicular chain would be reconstructed.

89

Attic Cholesteatoma

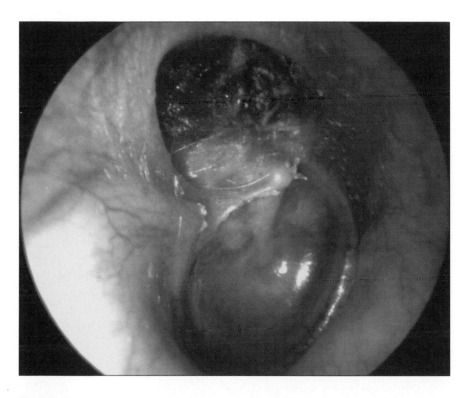

Fig 89–1

The otoscopic photograph is that of a right ear with attic cholesteatoma and normal pars tensa. The round defect in the posterior superior bony external auditory canal appears slightly smaller than the annular ring and is superior to it. The defect is filled with debris of desquamated epithelium and brown cerumen. The defect replaces bone of the external ear canal and extends into the epitympanum and probably the antrum and mastoid. The inferior boundary of this defect is the superior edge of the pars tensa, which is high-lighted by a white fold extending from the posterior, annular ring to the short process of the malleus. The long process of the malleus is normal as is all of the pars tensa. The normal lenticular process of the incus and stapes can be seen through the posterior superior quadrant of the pars tensa. The chorda tympani is visible as it courses over the incus and under the handle of the malleus. Treatment involves tympanoplasty with mastoidectomy and preservation of the posterior bony canal wall, pars tensa, and the integrity of the tympanum. The incus and head of the malleus are removed with the disease. The pars flaccida and canal skin over the defect are repaired with temporalis fascia and the entire mastoid cavity and epitympanum must be obliterated with bone paste to prevent recurrent cholesteatoma. Hearing is restored at a second-stage procedure through a speculum through the external auditory canal.

90

Attic Cholesteatoma and Tympanosclerosis

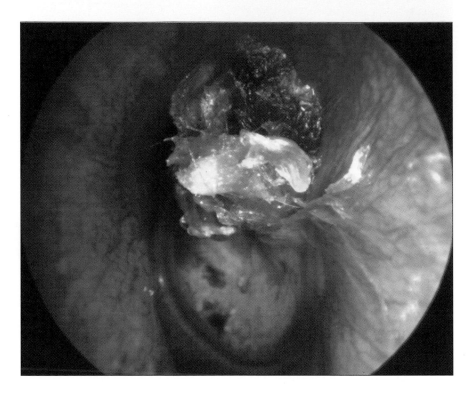

Fig 90–1

Two or more problems often are present in ears with chronic suppurative otitis media. This is an otoscopic view of a left ear with both attic cholesteatoma and tympanosclerosis of the pars tensa. It is likely that the tympanosclerosis is a longstanding problem and the attic cholesteatoma has developed more recently. There is no active infection but the expanding cholesteatoma, because of the accumulation of epithelial debris, represents potential risk of complication including facial paralysis, labyrinthine fistula, meningitis, and brain abscess. It represents a type VI chronic suppurative otitis media as described by the authors.[1] At the superior edge of the pars tensa there is a mass of yellow and white desquamated epithelium and brown cerumen exuding out of the attic into the external ear canal. The whitish-colored tympanosclerosis almost com-

pletely replaces the pars tensa and probably fixes the malleus, which can be seen in a vertical position in the center of the superior half of the pars tensa. The handle of the malleus and the umbo are outlined by red capillaries. Because the pars tensa is opaque, it is not possible to determine by otoscopic examination how far the cholesteatoma extends into the tympanum. Surgical treatment of this type of ear pathology requires a type VI myringoplasty, tympanoplasty, and mastoidectomy with removal of cholesteatoma as described by Pulec.[2] No preoperative medical treatment is required. In this case, the procedure begins by removal of the canal skin through a speculum with preservation of the vascular strip. The entire pars tensa is discarded and any cholesteatoma within the middle ear is removed. A postauricular incision is made and all cholesteatoma is removed from the mastoid and from the epitympanum. A disk of Silastic film may or may not be required to prevent adhesions in the middle ear. A tympanic membrane graft is accomplished and the entire mastoid and epitympanum are obliterated with bone paste in such a way that the dehiscent superior medial portion of the external auditory canal, which had been destroyed by the cholesteatoma, is reconstructed. Four to 6 months later, a second-stage tympanoplasty through the ear canal is used to remove the Silastic film and to recontruct hearing.

References

1. Pulec J, Deguine C. Classification of chronic suppurative otitis media. *Operative Tech Otolaryngol Head Neck Surg.* 1995;6(1):2–4.
2. Pulec J. A surgical system of management of chronic suppurative otitis media. *Operative Tech Otolaryngol Head Neck Surg.* 1995;6(1):5–16.

91

Attic Cholesteatoma With Facial Palsy

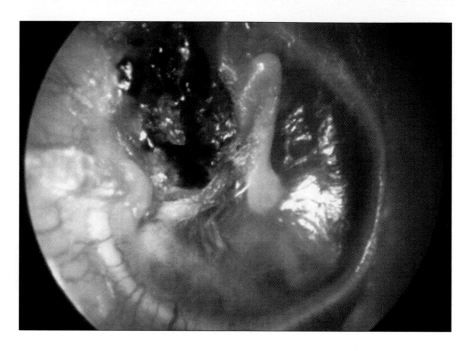

Fig 91–1

Complications of untreated attic cholesteatoma include facial palsy, labyrinthine fistulae, labyrinthitis, brain abscess, and meningitis. This is the otoscopic view of a right ear with attic cholesteatoma in a patient with slowly developing, partial (50%) facial palsy of 6 hours' duration. This is type IV chronic suppurative otitis media. The pars tensa is completely normal except for the posterior superior quadrant, which has been destroyed by the enlarging cholesteatoma. There is 3 mm of erosion of the posterior superior external auditory canal bone. The vertical cream-colored malleus occupies the center of the superior half of the pars tensa. The anterior pars flaccida and anterior epitympanum are free of disease. Through the translucent pars tensa the light-colored bone of the promontory is seen and, inferior to the umbo and posterior to the

promontory, the dark round window niche is seen. Several prominent red capillaries on the surface skin of the posterior inferior external auditory canal cross the annulus. The retracted pars flaccida has created an apparent perforation and the desquamating epithelium of the growing basement membrane forms an enlarging and destructive tumor. Within minutes of the first examination, using the operating microscope in the office, the interior of the cholesteatoma was removed to relieve pressure on the tympanic portion of the facial nerve. Facial palsy resolved within a few hours. The following day, an intact canal wall type IV tympanoplasty and mastoidectomy with bone paste obliteration was performed for definitive treatment. Hearing was restored by ossicular reconstruction 4 months later.

Atlas of Otoscopy

Attic Cholesteatoma and Polyp With a Blue Eardrum

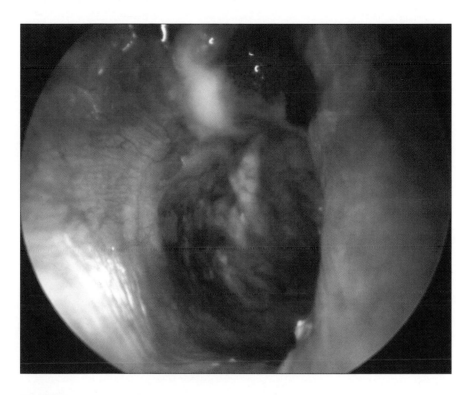

Fig 92–1

The otoscopic view is that of a right ear with an attic defect filled with cholesteatoma and a polyp. The handle of the malleus can be seen inferior to the polyp and the entire pars tensa is intact. The pars tensa has a dull, bluish color, commonly called "the blue eardrum." The blue color is caused by serous fluid stained with hemosiderin, usually from cholesterol granuloma. This case represents a type IV chronic suppurative otitis media, as described by the authors.[1] Although office treatment with an antibiotic steroid and steroid-containing eardrop used four times daily will often shrink the polyp and improve the infection, definitive treatment is surgical. The procedure to be performed for this type of disease is type IV: transcanal removal of attic cholesteatoma and mastoidectomy, as described by

Pulec.[2] The pars tensa is left untouched, all squamous epithelium of the cholesteatoma and of obstructing granulation tissue is removed, the posterior bony external auditory canal and the skin of the external auditory canal are left untouched with the exception of the area of the perforation; and after the perforation has been repaired with fascia, the entire epitympanum and mastoid is obliterated with bone paste. The serous fluid in the tympanum usually resolves with this treatment, but if it persists for more than 6 weeks after surgery, a myringotomy and ventilating button can be used. Reconstruction for hearing is done under a local anesthetic 6 months after the mastoidectomy using an approach through a speculum through the external auditory canal to perform a tympanomeatal flap.

References

1. Pulec J, Deguine C. Classification of chronic suppurative otitis media. *Operative Tech Otolaryngol Head Neck Surg.* 1995;6(1):2–4.

2. Pulec J. A surgical system of management of chronic suppurative otitis media. *Operative Tech Otolaryngol Head Neck Surg.* 1995;6(1):5–16.

93

Attic Cholesteatoma and Extensive Tympanosclerosis

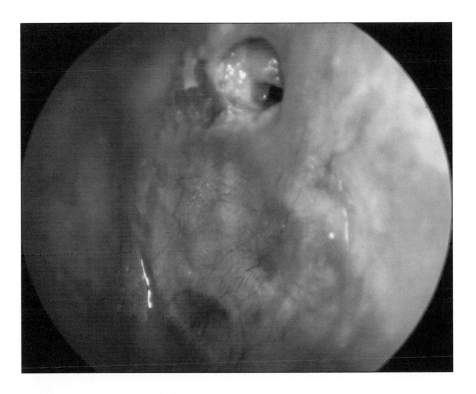

Fig 93–1

Attic cholesteatoma can appear in a variety of different ways, depending on the stage and development of the disease. This otoscopic view of a left ear demonstrates an uninfected attic cholesteatoma with a small opening through the pars flaccida, posterior to the short process and the neck of the malleus. There is relatively little debris within the retracted pars flaccida pouch. The anterior canal wall at the left third of the photograph appears rose-colored. A small area of inflammation suggesting early granulation tissue formation lies anterior to the short process of the malleus. The entire pars tensa is distorted with extensive tympanosclerosis. It is impossible to tell how far the squamous epithe-lium and cholesteatoma extend into the tympanum because the pars tensa is opaque. This ear has both an attic cholesteatoma and disease of the tympanum. It is a Pulec-Deguine type VI classification of chronic otitis media. Surgical treatment requires a Pulec type VI myringoplasty, tympanoplasty, and mastoidectomy with removal of cholesteatoma. Because of the attic cholesteatoma, definitive treatment includes obliteration of the epitympanum and mastoid with bone paste to prevent the recurrence of attic cholesteatoma. The entire procedure is done by preserving the bony external auditory canal. Secondary reconstruction of the ossicular chain after a period of healing for 6 months usually restores hearing.

Attic Cholesteatoma With Erosion of the Superior Bony Canal Wall

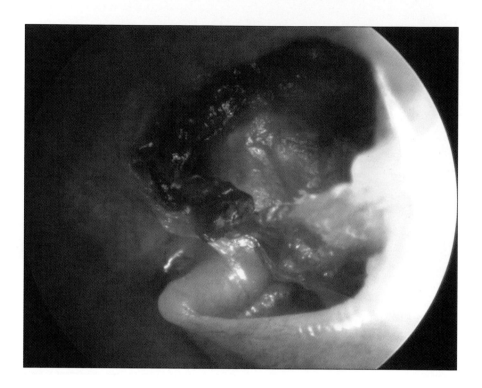

Fig 94–1

The otoscopic view demonstrates a close-up of the attic cholesteatoma in a left ear. There is no infection. The retracted pars tensa lining the cavity is filled with dead squamous epithelium and cerumen, which appears as a brownish, yellow mass. The constantly expanding mass of debris within the cholesteatoma has produced significant erosion of the superior bony external auditory canal. Only a small view of the otherwise normal pars tensa is seen at the lower edge of the photograph. The short process of the malleus is seen at the lower portion of the middle of the photograph and immediately to the right of the malleus is an extension of the cholesteatoma sac into the tympanum. This is type IV chronic suppurative otitis media, as described elsewhere by the authors.[1] Treatment requires a type IV transcanal removal of an attic cholesteatoma and mastoidectomy with obliteration of the epitympanum and mastoid to prevent *recurrent* attic cholesteatoma, as described by Pulec.[2] The procedure involves preservation of the posterior bony external auditory canal and total removal of cholesteatoma from the tympanum, epitympanum, and mastoid; excision of the perforation of the pars flaccida; and preservation of the normal part of the pars tensa. Secondary transcanal reconstruction of the ossicular chain for hearing is performed after 6 months.

References

1. Pulec J, Deguine C. Classification of chronic suppurative otitis media. *Operative Tech Otolaryngol Head Neck Surg.* 1995;6(1):2–4.
2. Pulec J. A surgical system of management of chronic suppurative otitis media. *Operative Tech Otolaryngol Head Neck Surg.* 1995;6(1):5–16.

95

Attic Cholesteatoma Producing a Natural Modified Radical Mastoidectomy

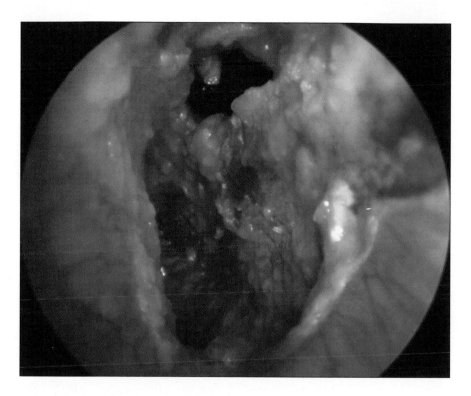

Fig 95–1

The otoscopic view is of a left ear demonstrating an intact pars tensa and an attic cholesteatoma that has destroyed a large portion of the posterior, superior external auditory canal so that it has an appearance of a surgically produced, modified radical mastoidectomy. The pars tensa is intact and the surface is covered with some moist epithelial debris, which appears in white patches. There is erythema surrounding the handle of the malleus. Immediately superior to the handle of the malleus within the attic defect at the superior part of the photograph is a dark area of clotted blood lying in the exposed epitympanum. To the right, a yellow patch of pus covers the medial wall of the naturally created mastoid cavity. This ear represents a Pulec-Deguine type IV chronic suppurative otitis media. Treatment is surgical, as it would be for a previously created modified radical mastoidectomy cavity. Treatment is a Pulec type IV tympanoplasty transcanal excision of attic cholesteatoma defect, mastoidectomy, tympanoplasty, obliteration of the cavity, and reconstruction of the external auditory canal with bone paste covered with fascia. Ossicular reconstruction is done after 6 months when the bony canal wall is healed with hard bone. Good hearing can usually be obtained.

Attic Cholesteatoma With Atelectasis

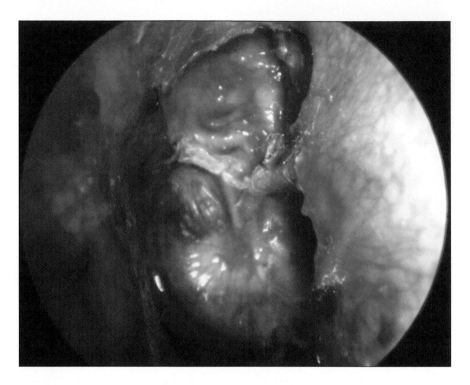

Fig 96–1

This is an otoscopic view of a left ear demonstrating an attic cholesteatoma with significant erosion of bone of the external auditory canal. At the top of the photograph, brownish green purulent debris is seen lining the attic defect. The pinkish, white vertical bone in the center of the photograph is the handle of the malleus. The head and neck of the malleus appear to be missing. The anterior half of the pars tensa is involved with tympanosclerosis. The posterior half of the pars tensa has only two layers and is retracted into the sinus tympani and suprapyramidal recess. The pars tensa gives the appearance of fluid within the tympanum. This is a type VI chronic suppurative otitis media, as described previously by the authors.[1] Surgical repair involves type VI myringoplasty, tympanoplasty, and mastoidectomy with removal of cholesteatoma and reconstruction of the bony defect in the external auditory canal by filling the epitympanum and mastoid with bone paste to prevent *recurrent* attic cholesteatoma, as described by Pulec.[2] Should serous fluid persist within the middle ear after the ear has healed, a ventilating tube through the new graft of the pars tensa may be required. Ossicular reconstruction to restore hearing can be performed after 6 months.

References

1. Pulec J, Deguine C. Classification of chronic suppurative otitis media. *Operative Tech Otolaryngol Head Neck Surg.* 1995;6(1):2–4.
2. Pulec J. A surgical system of management of chronic suppurative otitis media. *Operative Tech Otolaryngol Head Neck Surg.* 1995;6(1):5–16.

97

Attic Cholesteatoma in the Anterior Epitympanum

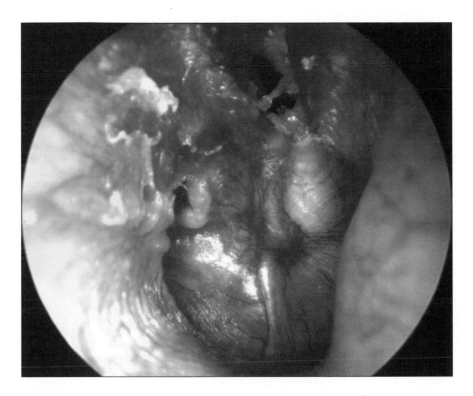

Fig 97–1

The otoscopic view is that of a right ear with an attic cholesteatoma originating anterior to the head and neck of the malleus. At the top of the photograph an opening is seen anterior to the malleus. There is no active infection and the ear is dry. There is marked erythema of the canal skin and along the handle of the malleus, which is vertical in the center of the photograph. To the right of the handle of the malleus, an extension of cholesteatoma can be seen through the translucent pars tensa. At the far right, the bulge of the anterior bony canal wall obscures the view of the anterior annulus. The anterior half of the pars tensa is otherwise normal. The posterior half of the pars tensa has had a perforation that has healed or has lost the fibrous layer through an immune reaction and is retracted onto the promontory, the stapes, and the incus. The intact stapes can be seen through this thin neomembrane. The lentic-ular process of the incus has been eroded and the remnant is seen near the capitulum of the stapes. This is an instance of Pulec-Deguine type VI chronic suppurative otitis media and requires a Pulec type VI myringoplasty, tympanoplasty, and mastoidectomy with removal of cholesteatoma.[1,2] The anterior canal wall skin is removed so that the anterior canal wall bulge can be removed to allow visualization of the anterior annulus. The posterior bony canal wall is left intact and the vascular strip of skin posteriorly is left undisturbed. The epitympanum and mastoid are obliterated with bone paste to prevent recurrence of the attic cholesteatoma. The tympanic membrane is grafted with fascia, perichondrium, or a homograft. Reconstruction of the ossicular chain for the restoration of hearing is performed through the external auditory canal under a local anesthetic after 6 months.

References

1. Pulec J, Deguine C. Classification of chronic suppurative otitis media. *Operative Tech Otolaryngol Head Neck Surg.* 1995;6(1):2–4.

2. Pulec J. A surgical system of management of chronic suppurative otitis media. *Operative Tech Otolaryngol Head Neck Surg.* 1995;6(1):5–16.

98

Attic Cholesteatoma With Extension into the Tympanum

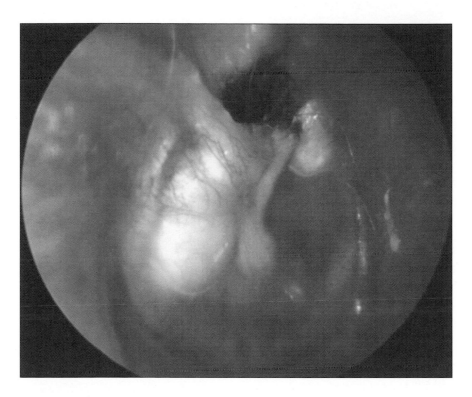

Fig 98–1

The otoscopic view is that of a right ear demonstrating a large attic defect. The handle of the malleus is vertical in the center of the photograph. The head and neck of the malleus and the incus are missing. The pars tensa is almost completely normal. A mass of cream-colored tissue anterior to the lateral process of the malleus is visible medial to the pars tensa. A globular pearl-appearing mass is seen pressing against the posterior portion of the pars tensa. This is an attic cholesteatoma extending inferiorly into the tympanum to the level of the round window. This is a Pulec-Deguine classification type IV chronic otitis media.[1] Treatment required is a Pulec type IV tympanoplasty and mastoidectomy.[2] The edges of the perforation must be excised. A generous tympanomeatal flap may be necessary to provide exposure to dissect the cholesteatoma from the tympanum. In most cases, the cholesteatoma and its basement membrane will separate easily from the

pars tensa, allowing the pars tensa to be preserved. Complete removal of the remaining cholesteatoma in the epitympanum, antrum, and mastoid is accomplished through a postauricular approach. The posterior bony external auditory canal is left unharmed and intact. The mastoid cavity and epitympanum must be obliterated with bone paste and the perforation is repaired with an underlay graft of fascia. Second-stage ossicular reconstruction is required after a healing period of at least 6 months.

References

1. Pulec J, Deguine C. Classification of chronic suppurative otitis media. *Operative Tech Otolaryngol Head Neck Surg.* 1995;6(1):2–4.
2. Pulec J. A surgical system of management of chronic suppurative otitis media. *Operative Tech Otolaryngol Head Neck Surg.* 1995;6(1):5–16.

99

Type V Chronic Suppurative Otitis Media

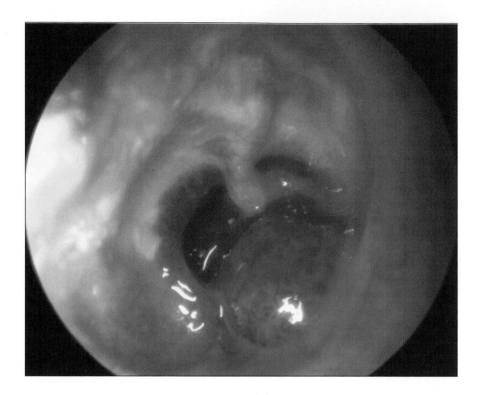

Fig 99–1

The otoscopic view is of a right ear that is acutely infected and draining thick, yellow pus. There is a 70% perforation of the pars tensa. The malleus appears to be grossly normal. The drum remnant has a rim of granulation tissue around the perforation and a large granulation tissue polyp protrudes through the anterior, inferior part of the perforation. This is a Pulec-Deguine type V chronic suppurative otitis media.[1] Treatment first involves systemic antibiotics and topical drops containing antibiotics and a steroid. In many cases, the ear can be made dry and the granulation tissue will resolve. In such cases, surgical treatment may involve a myringoplasty. When a reasonable trial of 2 or 3 weeks of medical therapy is unsuccessful in producing a dry ear, a type V Pulec tympanoplasty and mastoidectomy is performed.[2] The attic is left untouched.

Drainage is established through the facial recess from the mastoid to the tubotympanum. The pars tensa perforation is repaired with fascia. This conservative approach usually allows the infection to subside, the edematous polypoid mucosa obstructing the attic to heal, and in most cases, hearing to be restored to normal without the need for ossicular reconstruction. This type of ear infection represents 50% of cases requiring mastoidectomy.

References

1. Pulec J, Deguine C. Classification of chronic suppurative otitis media. *Operative Tech Otolaryngol Head Neck Surg.* 1995;6(1):2–4.
2. Pulec J. A surgical system of management of chronic suppurative otitis media. *Operative Tech Otolaryngol Head Neck Surg.* 1995;6(1):5–16.

100

Pars Tensa Perforation With Cholesteatoma

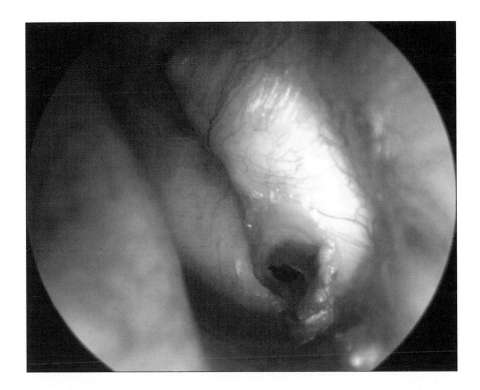

Fig 100–1

Cholesteatoma filling the posterior superior quadrant of the tympanum is often related to an attic cholesteatoma beginning with invagination of the pars flaccida. At first glance, the otoscopic view of this left tympanic membrane suggests the presence of an attic cholesteatoma. After careful study, however, the pars flaccida is seen to be intact and there is a perforation of the pars tensa at the inferior edge of the cholesteatoma near the annulus. At the superior edge of the photograph, the short process of the malleus and 1 mm of the long process can be seen in its normal position. Anterior to the manubrium of the malleus, the pars tensa is intact. The white cholesteatoma cyst is seen posterior to the manubrium of the malleus and fills the entire posterior tympanum. There is a perforation of the pars tensa at the inferior edge of this cholesteatoma and

it appears that the posterior half of the pars tensa has been replaced with a thin neomembrane through which the cholesteatoma cyst is seen. Anterior to the malleus, extension of the cholesteatoma can be seen through the translucent, otherwise normal, pars tensa. This case, most probably, represents a type III chronic suppurative otitis media, as described elsewhere by the authors.[1] There is a 90% probability that the cholesteatoma is confined to the tympanum and could be removed completely by a transcanal approach through a speculum as described as a type III myringoplasty and tympanoplasty combined by Pulec.[2] There is, however, a possibility that the cholesteatoma extends into the epitympanum, deeply into the facial recess, or into an anatomically unusually deep sinus tympani (type VI chronic suppurative otitis media), which would require an intact canal wall mastoidectomy to accomplish complete removal. With either of these situations, no preoperative treatment is required and conventional imaging available today is not helpful in determining whether a postauricular incision will be required. The case is best managed by informing the patient and by shaving the hair and draping the ear in preparation for a postauricular procedure. The transcanal approach will be satisfactory for most cases, but if the cholesteatoma cannot be completely removed, a postauricular approach can then be accomplished. Either local or general anesthesia can be used, depending on the time required for the surgery. Silastic film is used to prevent adhesions. Second-stage reconstruction of hearing is done after 4 months.

References

1. Pulec JL, Deguine C. Classification of chronic suppurative otitis media. *Operative Tech Otolaryngol Head Neck Surg.* 1995;6(1):2–4.
2. Pulec JL. A surgical system of management of chrnoic suppurative otitis media. *Operative Tech Otolaryngol Head Neck Surg.* 1995;6(1):5–16.

101

Chronic Suppurative Otitis Media With Tympanosclerosis and Cholesteatoma

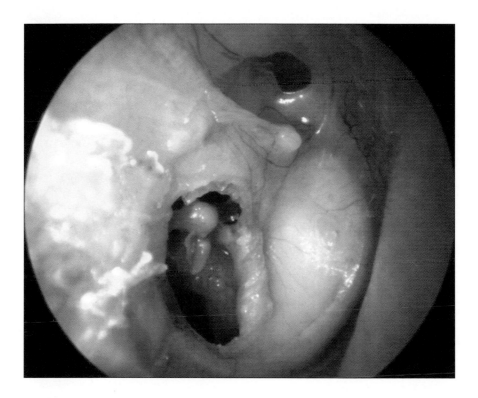

Fig 101–1

The otoscopic view is that of a right ear with chronic suppurative otitis media of the Pulec-Deguine classification type VI.[1] Observation immediately discloses five pathologic conditions:

1. There is a 45% marginal perforation of the posterior part of the pars tensa.
2. The stapes can be seen through the perforation. with loss of the lenticular process of the incus.
3. The anterior part of the pars tensa is involved in opaque, cream-colored tympanosclerosis.
4. A small attic perforation is present anterior to the malleus.
5. Squamous epithelium is seen extending into the middle ear through the pars tensa perforation as a combination of rolls of yellow material at the anterior edge of the perforation and is jagged, white, and almost sawtooth in appearance around the superior and inferior edges of the pars tensa perforation.

It is likely that the surgeon will find squamous epithelium covering the medial surface of the pars tensa and extending into the facial recess and part of the tympanum. An attic cholesteatoma is likely, which may or may not extend into the mastoid. Treatment is by Pulec type VI tympanoplasty and mastoidectomy with preservation of the bony external auditory canal followed in 6 months by second-stage reconstruction of the ossicular chain through the ear canal.[2]

References

1. Pulec JL, Deguine C. Classification of chronic suppurative otitis media. *Operative Tech Head Neck Surg.* 1995;6(1):2–4.
2. Pulec JL. A surgical system of management of chronic suppurative otitis media. *Operative Tech Head Neck Surg.* 1995;6(1):5–16.

102

Tuberculous Chronic Otitis Media

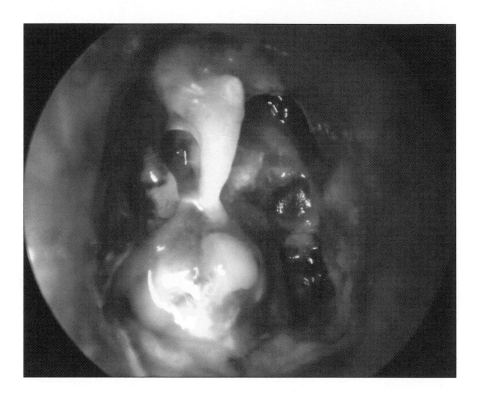

Fig 102–1

The otoscopic view is that of a right ear in a 5-year-old girl. There is a total perforation of the pars tensa with purulent otorrhea covering the promontory and floor of the ear canal. The malleus is cream-colored, and extends vertically from the upper portion of the photo. No pars tensa is attached. The pars flaccida is retracted. There is the appearance of the incus and stapes in the left upper quadrant, although a clear view is not possible because of the thick pus covering these structures. Tuberculous as the etiology of chronic suppurative otitis media is uncommonly seen in a modern otologic practice. For this reason it is sometimes initially undiagnosed and the surgeon is surprised to find that infection persists following tympanoplasty and mastoidectomy. The diagnosis is confirmed by bacteriologic smear and culture. It is best to treat the patient systematically until active otorrhea subsides. After the ear becomes dry with systemic treatment and local cleansing, tympanoplasty and mastoidectomy can provide permanent closure of the tympanic membrane and restoration of hearing.

103

Tuberculous Chronic Otitis Media

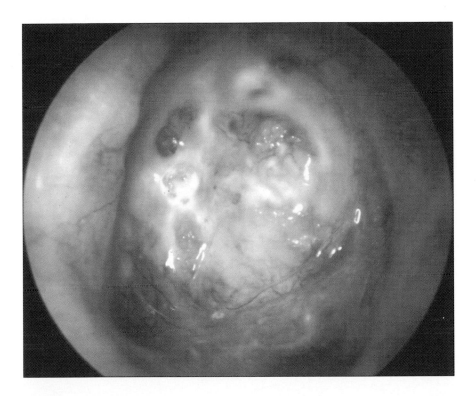

Fig 103–1

The otoscopic view is that of the left ear of the same 5-year-old girl described in the previous chapter. With the exception of the external auditory canal and the suggestion of an annulus, no landmarks are visible. The medial wall of the tympanum is covered with pale-pink-colored granulation tissue and mucopus. Stain for acid-fast bacilli and culture are needed to confirm the diagnosis of tuberculous otitis media.

104

Chronic Suppurative Otitis Media: Type I

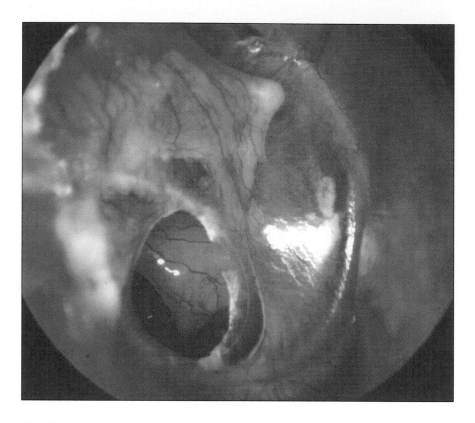

Fig 104–1

The otoscopic view is that of a right ear demonstrating a dry posterior-inferior 25% perforation of the pars tensa. The smooth, glistening mucosa of the promontory and the dark oval area of the round window niche are seen through the left of the perforation. The very small cosmetic patch of tympanosclerosis is in the pars tensa near the anterior annulus.

105

Right Postoperative Type I Tympanoplasty

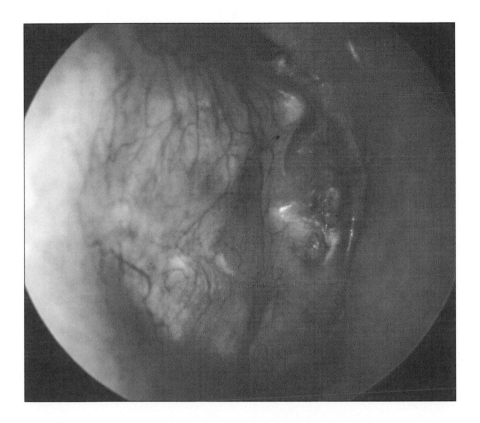

Fig 105–1

This otoscopic view is of the same right ear shown in Chapter 104 1 year after successful tympanoplasty. The procedure was performed through the external auditory canal using an underlay fascia graft. The anterior portion of the tympanic membrane and ear canal appear the same as the preoperative view. The posterior half of the pars tensa has a thickened, healed graft with prominent blood vessels visible.

106

Type I Chronic Suppurative Otitis Media

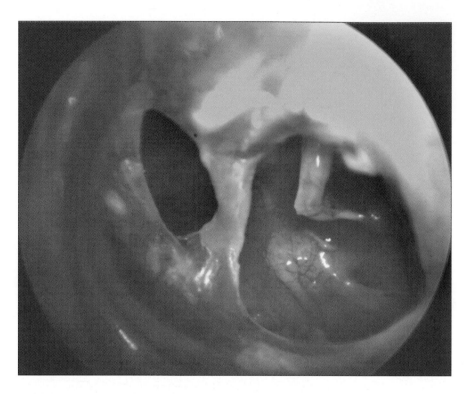

Fig 106–1

Preoperative view of a left ear demonstrating two dry perforations of the pars tensa. A remnant of the pars tensa is attached to the umbo of the malleus and occupies the anterior-inferior quadrant. A perforation of the pars tensa is in the anterior-superior quadrant and the entire posterior half of the tympanic membrane is involved with a second perforation. The incus, stapes, and malleus appear normal. There is no evidence of cholesteatoma or squamous epithelium in the middle ear.

107

Postoperative, Healed Type I Tympanoplasty

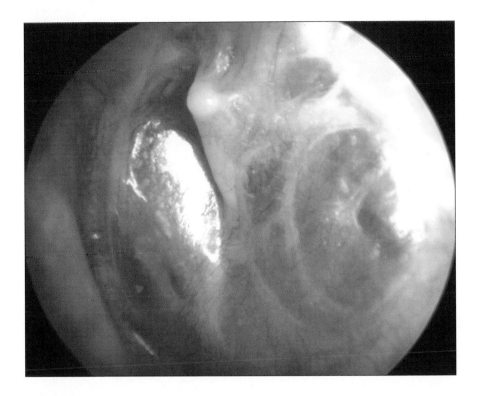

Fig 107–1

This is the same left ear shown in the last chapter 1 year following type I tympanoplasty. A underlay fascia graft was used to reconstruct the entire pars tensa. Hearing was restored. Note the scarring of the pars tensa with partial loss of normal contour and landmarks. The appearance is typical of a postoperative fascia graft tympanoplasty.

Type I Chronic Suppurative Otitis Media

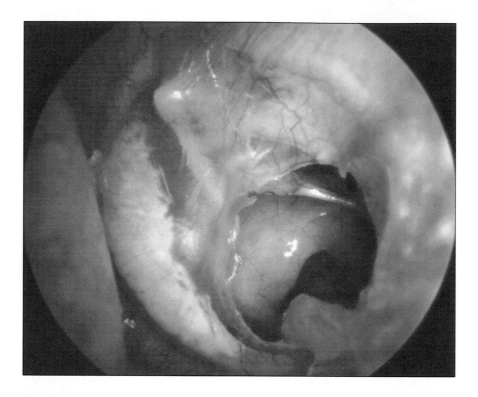

Fig 108–1

The otoscopic view is that of a left ear with a dry posterior-inferior perforation of the pars tensa. A semilunar area of white tympanosclerosis is in the anterior tympanic remnant. The long process of the malleus and the short process are clearly seen. Through the perforation the capitulum of the stapes and, posterior to that, the stapedius tendon can be seen. Inferior to the stapes is the glistening mucous membrane covering the normal promontory and posterior to the promontory is the dark depression of the round window niche.

109

Postoperative Type I Tympanoplasty

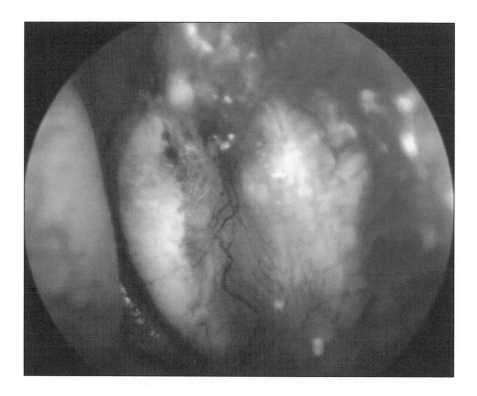

Fig 109–1

The otoscopic view is of the same left ear shown in the last chapter 1 year following successful tympanoplasty. An underlay technique using fascia was used. Many of the landmarks have been lost, although the same unchanged tympanosclerosis and anterior pars tensa can be observed. The posterior half of the pars tensa is replaced with a thickened fascia graft. There is no perforation. Hearing was restored to normal.

SECTION VIII

Trauma

110

Traumatic Perforation: Concussion

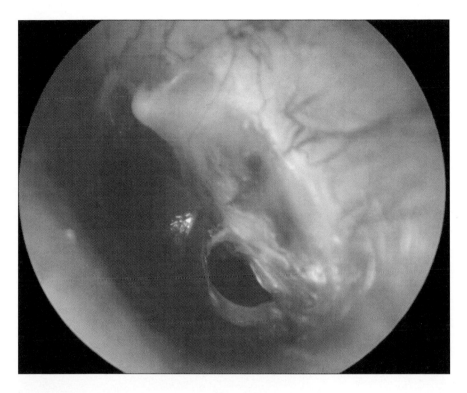

Fig 110–1

The otoscopic view is that of a left ear of a patient 4 days after being struck on the ear with a cupped hand. This view demonstrates a 20% dry perforation in the inferior portion of pars tensa. The remainder of the ear is normal. The edges of the torn pars tensa can be seen folded under the medial surface of the tympanic membrane perforation. There is no infection or blood clot. The patient complained of ringing, high-pitched tinnitus, which subsided 1 day after the injury, and a persistent feeling of fullness in the ear. Management includes the performance of an audiometric examination for pure tone and speech discrimination. Ninety percent of traumatic perforations of the tympanic membrane will heal spontaneously within 4 weeks. Myringoplasty can be performed on ears that fail to heal after 4 weeks. The usual success rate is 95%. No surgery should be performed before 4 weeks. The patient should be instructed to keep water out of the ear and to return for treatment of any otorrhea.

111
Traumatic Perforation: Spontaneous Healing

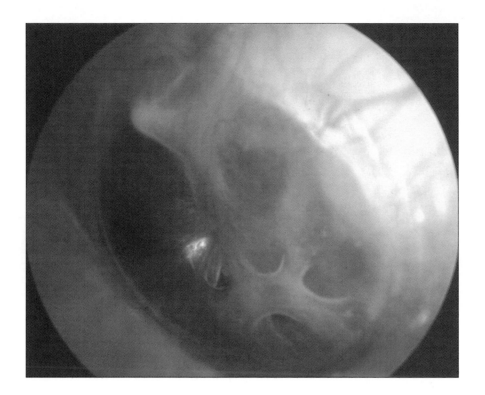

Fig 111–1

The otoscopic view is the same left ear seen in the previous chapter 1 month after the injury. Healing is complete and there is only a scar in the area of the previous perforation. The pars tensa is intact. The chorda tympani is seen through the pars tensa at the posterior superior quadrant of the tympanic membrane as well as the incus extending in a vertical direction at the posterior edge of the chorda tympani.

112

Traumatic Perforation: Q-tip Injury

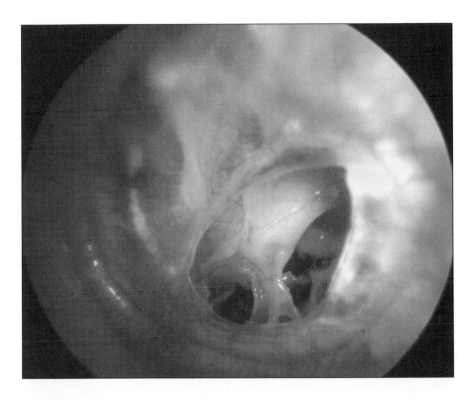

Fig 112–1

The otoscopic view is that of a left ear with a 30% dry perforation of the posterior inferior part of the pars tensa. The malleus and anterior pars tensa are normal. The promontory, hypotympanum, and round window niche are visible through the perforation.

The injury is common and occurs when a patient cleans or scratches the ear and accidentally drives the Q-tip through the tympanic membrane. Fortunately in this case the stapes was not dislocated which can result in vertigo, tinnitus, and permanent hearing loss.

113

Traumatic Perforation: Spontaneous Healing After 3 Months

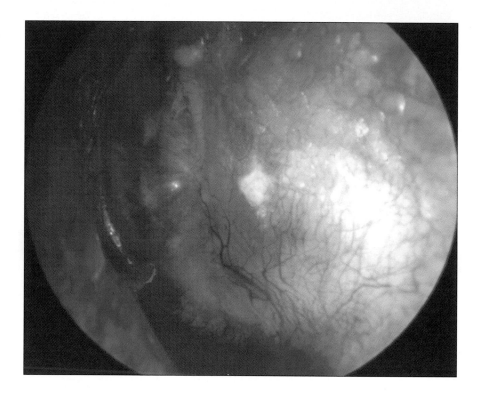

Fig 113–1

The otoscopic view is of the same left ear seen in the previous chapter 3 months after injury. Although the area of the healed perforation is slightly thickened, the tympanic membrane appears surprisingly normal. A minority of perforated tympanic membranes will heal after 1 month, those that do are usually large perforations that can be seen to be progressively healing at each follow-up examination.

114

Traumatic Perforation: Blast Injury

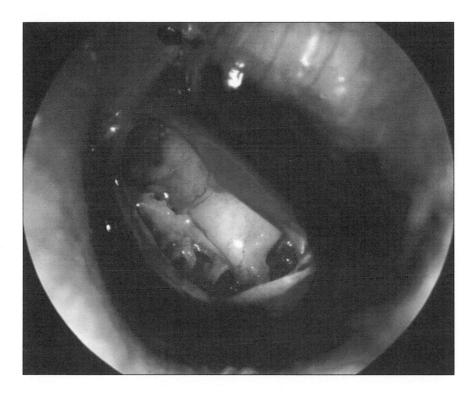

Fig 114–1

The otoscopic view is of the left ear of a patient who sustained a blast injury as the result of an industrial explosion. There is a 50% perforation of the anterior inferior portion of the tympanic membrane. Dark dry blood surrounds the perforation and there is bright red blood on the superior edge of the perforation. The round window niche, promontory, hypotympanum, and protympanum are seen through the perforation.

115

Healed Traumatic Perforation

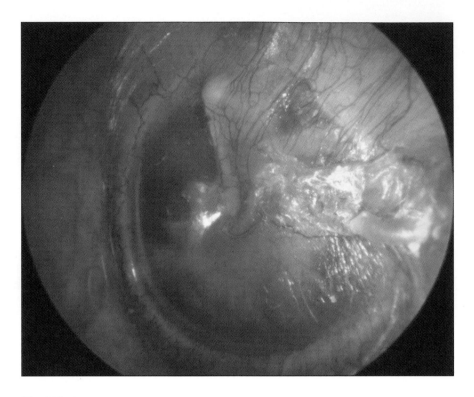

Fig 115–1

The accompanying otoscopic view is of the tympanic membrane of a left ear that sustained a large, traumatic perforation. The membrane appears in the photograph as it looked after 3 months of observation and complete spontaneous postinjury healing. The entire fibrous annulus can be seen, with an obvious area of demarcation along the fibrous annulus where the new tympanic membrane has healed with two layers. The fibrous layer is missing or has contracted into a white scar near the umbo. The short process of the malleus is the cream-colored 2-mm mass at the center of the superior portion of the tympanic membrane, extending inferiorly to the short process of the malleus. Anteriorly, the dark shadow of the tubotympanum can be seen. Posteriorly, lateral to the tympanic membrane, is a small, yellow mass of cerumen and desquamated epithelium, a common finding shortly after a perforation has healed. The tympanic membrane is intact and in a normal position, and the tympanum is well aerated.

Since 90% of traumatic perforations heal spontaneously within 1 to 3 months, surgical repair is normally withheld until 3 months have passed without spontaneous healing. The patient should be instructed to keep water out of the ear during this time, and any concurrent infection should be treated with systemic antibiotics and an ear drop containing an antibiotic and a steroid.

116

Hemotympanum

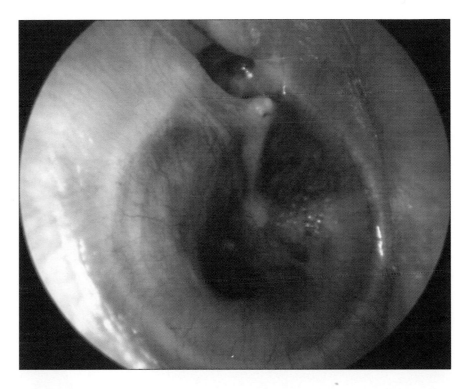

Fig 116–1

The dark blue, almost black color of an intact tympanic membrane indicates a tympanum filled with blood. In most cases, when associated with a history of trauma, it is pathognomonic of a temporal bone fracture. It may be associated with a conductive or sensorineural hearing loss, with or without vestibular involvement. Rarely, hemotympanum is caused by hemorrhage into the ear due to leukemia or as a result of the use of anticoagulants. Hemotympanum may be associated with hemoptysis as can be seen in advanced tuberculosis. Differential diagnosis includes the blue eardrum and cholesterol granuloma. Treatment of hemotympanum itself is conservative. Prophylactic antibiotics are often given to prevent infection. The condition usually resolves spontaneously within 4 weeks. If serous otitis media persists after 1 month, myringotomy and insertion of a ventilating tube for a few weeks may be needed.

117

Temporal Bone Fracture
With Displacement

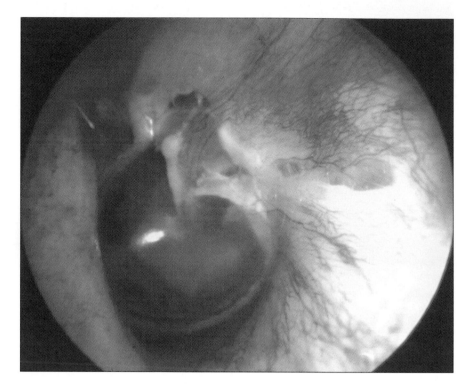

Fig 117–1

The otoscopic view is that of a left ear demonstrating a healed temporal bone fracture. Displacement of the posterior-superior bony external auditory canal and scarring of the posterior-superior tympanic membrane is demonstrated. A fracture is seen horizontal to the area of the incus and a second fracture is seen immediately anterior and superior to the short process of the malleus. The incus and stapes can be seen at the upper edge of the normal part of the pars tensa. This patient had a conductive hearing loss caused by dislocation and fixation of the incus. A Wehrs hydroxyapatite prosthesis was used to reconstruct the ossicular chain between the mobile malleus and the mobile capitulum of the stapes.

118

Old Temporal Bone Fracture

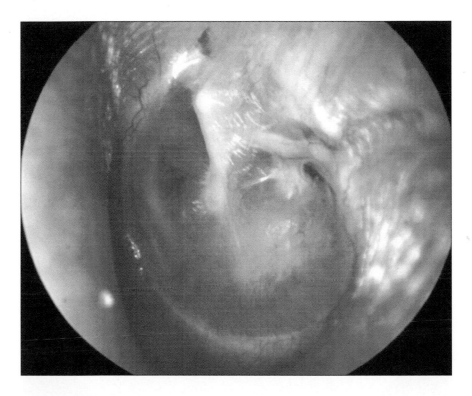

Fig 118–1

The otoscopic view is that of a left ear demonstrating evidence of a basilar skull fracture and two fractures of the temporal bone visible through the external auditory canal. The entire pars tensa is intact but there is an adhesion of the tympanic membrane to the incus. The malleus appears to be slightly anterior to its normal position. The chorda tympani is seen horizontally extending from near the short process of the malleus to the bone inferior to the posterior fracture. Fracture of the temporal bone can be seen immediately superior to the stapes and chorda tympani. A second fracture is seen anterior to the short process of the malleus. Despite the obvious fractures and myringostapedopexy, hearing was near-normal and no treatment was required.

119

Temporal Bone Fracture With Tympanic Membrane Perforation and Hemorrhage

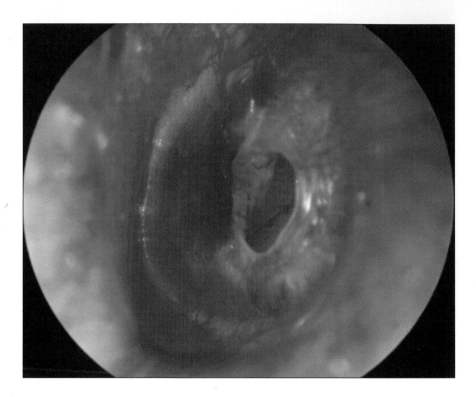

Fig 119–1

The otoscopic view is that of a left ear demonstrating an elliptical perforation immediately posterior to the malleus and hemorrhage involving the anterior portion of the pars tensa. This patient sustained a temporal bone fracture with perforation and bleeding. The tympanic membrane completely healed spontaneously after 4 weeks and required no treatment. Immediate treatment involves antibiotics to prevent secondary infection and the patient is advised to prevent water from entering the ear. Ninety percent of traumatic perforations will heal spontaneously. Should a perforation persist after 4 to 6 weeks, myringoplasty or tympanoplasty can be performed, which should be 95% successful.

120

Temporal Bone Fracture Following Spontaneous Healing

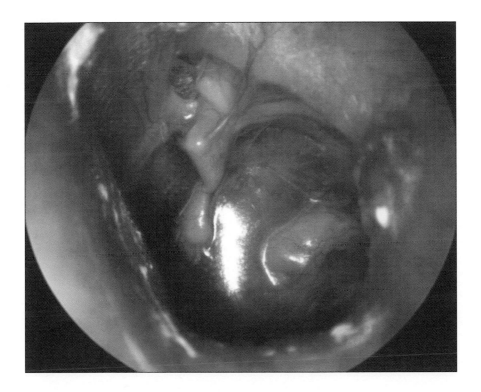

Fig 120–1

The otoscopic view is that of the same left ear seen in the previous chapter 6 weeks following injury. The posterior-superior perforation and damage to the posterior-superior canal wall has completely healed, and with the exception of the fracture site represented by a small jagged line at the posterior-superior edge of the photograph, the ear otherwise appears normal. Conductive hearing loss proved to be caused by a dislocation of the incus. Tympanoplasty by use of a tympanomeatal flap and placement of a Wehr's hydroxyapatite prosthesis resulted in successful restoration of hearing.

121

Temporal Bone Fracture With Conductive Hearing Loss

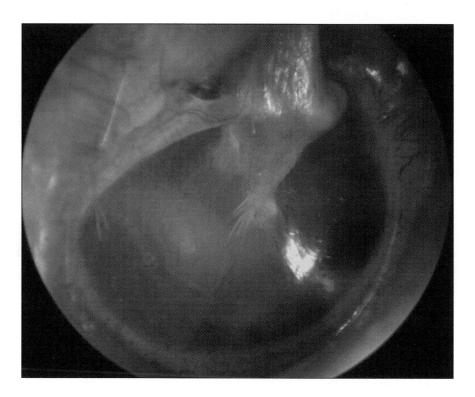

Fig 121–1

The otoscopic photograph is of the right ear and represents the effects of head trauma with temporal bone fracture. There is no evidence of infection, serous fluid, or hemotympanum. The pars tensa of the tympanic membrane is intact but the posterior-superior bony annulus is disrupted and dislocated by a fracture. The incus can be seen through the translucent pars tensa. The incus has been dislocated and the long process is in contact with the pars tensa. The lenticular process is detached from the capitulum of the stapes. This patient has a conductive hearing loss due to an ossicular discontinuity. Hearing can be restored by transcanal tympanoplasty performed as an outpatient with local anesthesia.

122

Obscure Temporal Bone Fracture With Conductive Hearing Loss

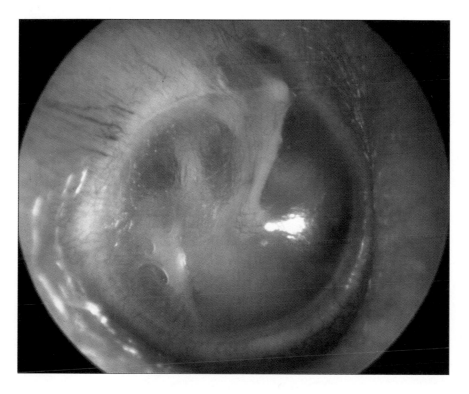

Fig 122–1

This otoscopic photograph demonstrates the right ear of patient who sustained a basilar skull fracture and fracture of the temporal bone many years before. The ear has been dry and free of any complaint with the exception of a 50-dB conductive hearing loss. There is minimal evidence of temporal bone fracture at the superior part of the annular ring along the notch of Rivinus. There is a healed posterior inferior perforation of the pars tensa which has an opaque scar. The long handle of the malleus is in the normal position. The incus is in a normal position. The stapes can be seen through the translucent pars tensa. Treatment involves tympanoplasty performed through the external auditory canal on an elective basis.

123

Old Temporal Bone Fracture With Dislocation of the Incus

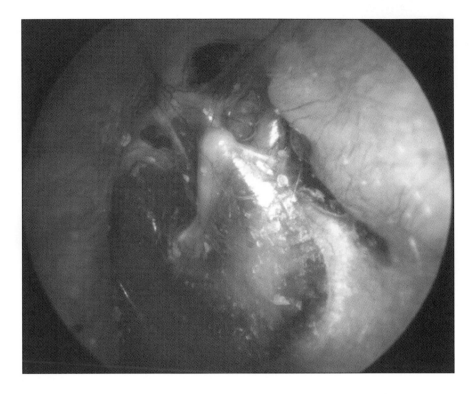

Fig 123–1

The otoscopic photograph is that of the left ear of a 15-year-old boy who gave a history of having a left conductive hearing loss since the age of 3½ years when he fell down a staircase. The pars tensa is intact and normal with a normal handle of the malleus. There is an obvious fracture extending from the superior external auditory canal near the annulus toward the posterior-superior part of the external auditory canal. A portion of bone in the superior bony canal wall is missing or dislocated. The body of the incus can be seen through the translucent pars tensa and it is dislocated inferiorly to a position lateral to the round window. Treatment involves tympanoplasty performed through the external auditory canal to reconstruct the ossicular chain.

124

Temporal Bone Fracture With Dislocation of the Incus

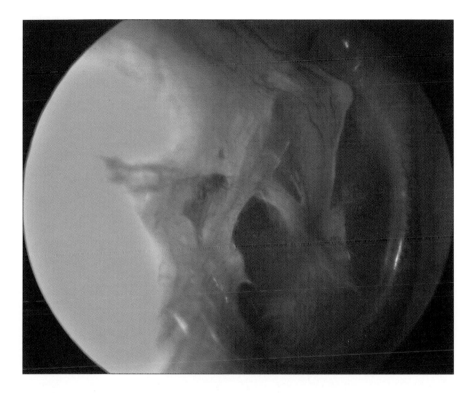

Fig 124–1

The otoscopic photograph is that of a right ear and represents the effect of head trauma with temporal bone fracture. The patient had no otorrhea, vertigo, or facial paralysis following head trauma. A conductive hearing loss occurred immediately after the trauma and has not improved with time. Two features are evident. There is a prominent fracture with dislocation extending along the posterior-superior bony external auditory canal. The pars tensa and pars flaccida are both intact. The long process of the incus can be seen through the tympanic membrane and is dislocated inferiorly. Restoration of hearing by tympanoplasty through the ear canal is performed on an elective basis.

125

Temporal Bone Fracture With Displacement of Bone

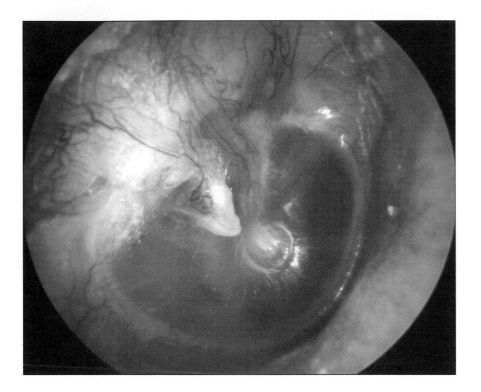

Fig 125–1

The otoscopic view is that of a right ear following healing after temporal bone fracture. The pars tensa is intact but is adherent to a dislocated incus and capitulum of the stapes. The malleus is in its normal position. The posterior-superior external auditory canal wall is dislocated and displaced into the external auditory canal. A large conductive hearing loss was the result of a dislocated incus and fractured crura. Ossicular reconstruction was required to restore normal hearing. In cases of this sort, it is often necessary to remove some of the displaced bone of the posterior ear canal to restore a normal contour and provide space for the reconstruction of the ossicular chain.

Traumatic Dislocation of the Incus

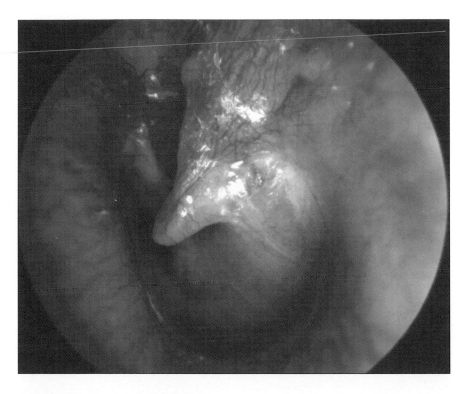

Fig 126–1

The otoscopic view is that of a left ear demonstrating an intact pars tensa and pars flaccida with the long process of the incus protruding through the pars tensa immediately posterior to the handle of the malleus near the umbo. Displacement of the bone of the external auditory canal indicative of a temporal bone fracture can be seen by the medial displacement with an apparent groove in the bone anterior to the short process of the malleus. The skin posterior to the short process of the malleus appears to be bulging from healing scar tissue. The white chorda tympani can be seen through the translucent pars tensa at the posterior-superior edge of the pars tensa near the bony annulus. The long process of the incus protrudes approximately 3 mm lateral to the pars tensa with healed squamous epithelium over its surface. Surgical repair is indicated to correct the conductive hearing loss by the use of a transcanal approach with the placement of a total occisular replacement prosthesis (TORP) or a partial ossicular replacement prosthesis (PORP) between the handle of the malleus or the tympanic membrane and the stapes capitulum or footplate.

127

Temporal Bone Fracture Post-tympanoplasty

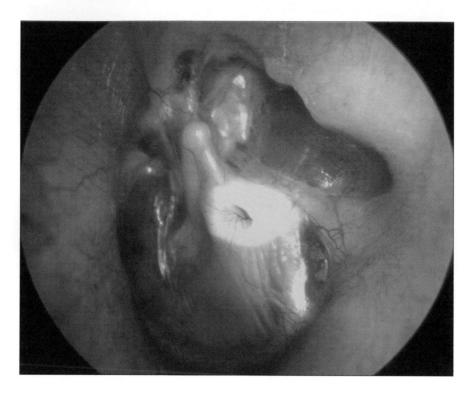

Fig 127–1

The otoscopic photograph is that of a left ear after complete healing of tympanoplasty for reconstruction of the ossicular chain using a Wehrs incus replacement prosthesis. The pars tensa is intact and normal. A hydroxyapatite incus replacement prosthesis can be seen medially posterior to the handle of the malleus through the translucent pars tensa. The chorda tympani passes superior to the prosthesis. A significant portion of bone of the posterior-superior bony canal wall is missing, which allows the pars flaccida to be retracted over the head and neck of the malleus, the tympanic portion of the facial nerve, and into the epitympanum. The tympanic portion of the fallopian canal appears as a pink, almost erythematous tube immediately superior and medial to the chorda tympani. Tympanoplasty surgery resulted in closure of the air-bone gap to less than 10 dB.

128

A Dislocated Incus Protruding Through a Traumatic Perforation*

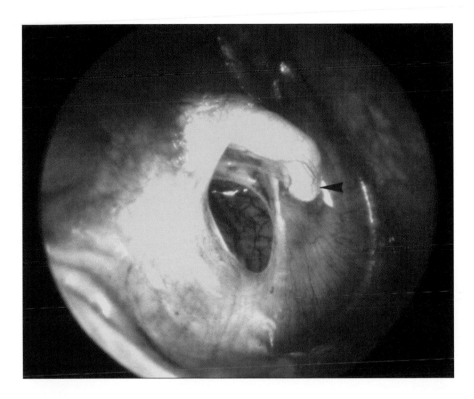

Fig 128–1

The otoscopic photograph of this right ear represents the consequence of a temporal bone fracture. This 41-year-old man had sustained a head injury after falling from a scaffold. He complained of right-sided hearing loss and delayed onset of facial weakness. Examination confirmed a central perforation of the pars tensa and partial paralysis of the right facial nerve. The middle ear contained a blood clot. A computed tomography scan of the brain and temporal bone showed a longitudinal fracture of the right temporal bone traversing the mastoid cavity, middle ear, and the petrous apex. The ossicular chain of the right ear was disrupted. Three weeks later his facial function had returned to normal; however, a pure-tone audiogram showed a 60 dB air-bone gap in this ear. Examination revealed a dislocated incus, with the long process (arrow)

protruding through the perforation of the pars tensa.

Exploratory tympanotomy showed that the dislocated incus was fixed in the attic and the malleus was missing. The stapes was intact and mobile. To facilitate the grafting of the perforated drum, the long process of the incus was excised. A Pulec Type II tympanoplasty was successfully performed and, 4 months later, the patient underwent an ossiculoplasty utilizing a partial ossicular replacement

*This chapter was contributed by Peter K.M. Ku, FRCS (Ed), Martin W. Pak, FRCS(Ed) and Charles A. van Hasselt, FRS(SA), MMed(Otol), Division of Otorhinolaryngology, The Chinese University of Hong Kong, Prince of Wales Hospital, Shatin, New Territories, Hong Kong.

prosthesis with reinforcement of the drum with a tragal cartilage graft. The patient noticed a dramatic improvement in hearing and the follow-up audiogram revealed a narrowing of the air-bone gap to 10 dB at 500 Hz, 1 kHz, and 2 kHz.

SECTION IX

Iatrogenic Disease

Epithelial Pearl Following Myringoplasty

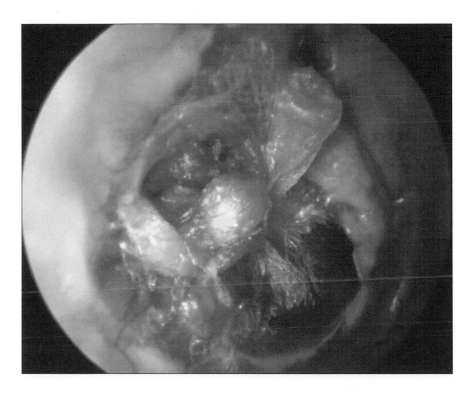

Fig 129–1

The otoscopic view is of a right ear that has had a myringoplasty and has developed an epithelial pearl on the surface of the tympanic membrane graft. The long process of the malleus can be seen descending from the middle of the superior edge of the tympanic membrane. A white 3-mm epithelial pearl lies on the lateral surface of the tympanic membrane graft immediately posterior and inferior to the umbo. There is a mass of epithelial debris posterior to the pearl. Tympanosclerosis is seen as a semilunar whitish material within the tympanic membrane graft lying near the anterior-inferior annulus and near the posterior annulus. The remainder of the pars tensa is thin and translucent. Epithelial cysts develop as the result of imperfect surgical technique when a fragment of squamous epithelium is covered or folded under the graft. When these cysts appear lateral to the graft, they can usually be eliminated by marsupializing them with a sharp needle without anesthesia in the office. Careful follow-up examination is required.

130

A "String of Pearls"*

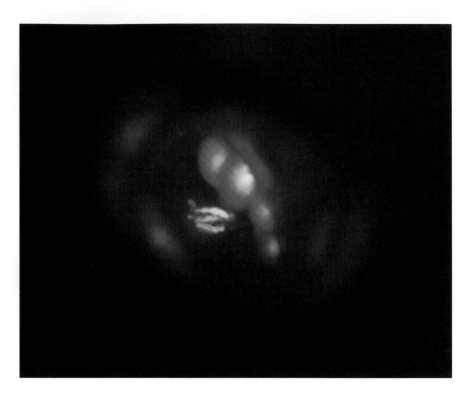

Fig 130–1

The otoscopic photograph illustrates the unusual healing phenomenon that occurred following a left middle-ear infection. The patient was a 3-year-old child examined by her pediatrician because of acute left otitis media. Despite appropriate oral antibiotic therapy, she continued to have ear pain. One morning she awakened with drainage from her left ear and the pain gone. Reexamination by her pediatrician revealed a central left TM perforation. She was referred for an otologic examination. There was a simple TM perforation noted. The margins were frayed. Under the microscope an attempt was made to reapproximate the margins of the perforation. Two weeks later when she was reexamined, the perforation was no longer present, but instead, five distinct contiguous encapsulated cholesteatoma pearls were observed on the lateral surface of the left eardrum. Because of her age, she was brought to the outpatient surgical unit. Under microscopic examination each of the five intratympanic cholesteatoma pearls was removed intact. Gelfoam was placed over the epithelial layer defect. The lateral epithelial layer eventually healed over with an intact drum and with at least a double layer membrane where the previous perforation had been. She had no auditory deficit and no further therapy was required.

*Chapter contributed by Joseph R. DiBartolomeo, MD, Santa Barbara, California.

131

Lateralization of Fascia Graft Myringoplasty

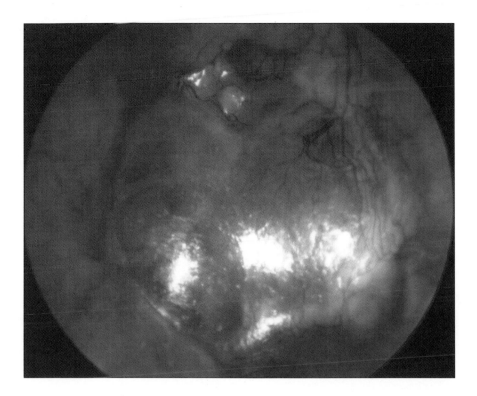

Fig 131–1

The otoscopic view is of a left ear of a 42-year-old man 9 years after fascia graft myringoplasty. The tympanic membrane graft is thin, translucent, and the tympanum is well aerated. There is no perforation or infection. There are no notable landmarks in the tympanic membrane graft. The membrane has a concave appearance with lateralization of the edges where it should have remained at the annulus. At the superior edge of the photograph, the white, short process of the malleus can be seen. Inferior to this, there is the hint of the long process of the malleus, which appears to be medial to, but not attached to, the tympanic membrane graft. Lateralization of the graft occurred despite the fact that the graft was placed under the handle of the malleus at the time of initial surgery. A conductive hearing loss of 15 dB was the result. Surgeons have used various modifications of technique to avoid or minimize movement of a fascia graft laterally and detachment from the handle of the malleus. Useful methods include placement of the fascia graft medial to the handle of the malleus and placement of the edges of the fascia medial to the tympanic membrane remnant or medial to the anterior and inferior portions of the fibrous annulus. The problem of lateral healing does not occur when canal skin and periosteum are used alone or with a homograft tympanic membrane.

132

Poorly Performed Modified Radical Mastoidectomy

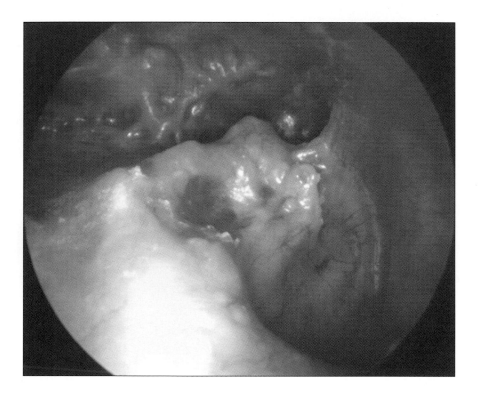

Fig 132–1

The otoscopic view is that of a right ear with a modified radical mastoidectomy. The anterior external auditory canal and inferior external auditory canal are present. The pars tensa, malleus, and incus are visible and were left untouched. The pars tensa is thickened with tympanosclerosis and there is the suggestion of serous fluid within the tympanum. The chorda tympani crosses from the posterior canaliculus anteriorly lateral to the incus and medial to the malleus. The superior and posterior external auditory canal has been previously removed and the cavity is lined with a very thin layer of squamous epithelium. The cavity contains many partially uncovered mastoid air cells and is the source of recurring accumulation of epithelial debris leading to a foul-smelling discharge. At the anterior-superior edge of the epitympanum, the membrane is thin and appears to seal the middle ear from the cavity. The Bondi modified radical mastoidectomy was developed in the 19th century to treat attic cholesteatoma by exterioration to make the ear "safe" and still preserve middle-ear structures and hearing. Modern tympanoplasty techniques have made this operation obsolete.

133

Radical Mastoidectomy Cavity Infected With Otomycosis

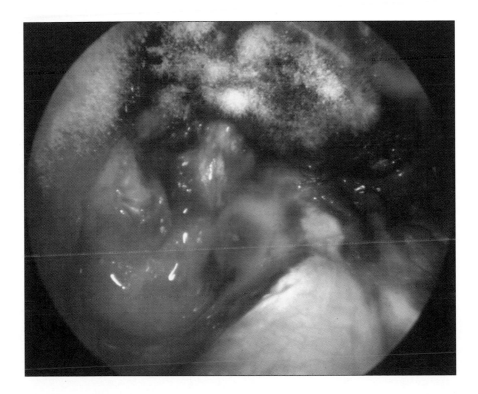

Fig 133–1

Radical mastoidectomy cavities, even when properly created, frequently have recurrent or persistent otorrhea. The otoscopic view is that of a left ear of a patient who has had a radical mastoidectomy. The surgeon had performed a meatoplasty, resulting in a large, cosmetically unpleasing external auditory canal. There is a foul-smelling discharge covering and obscuring the anatomy. In the superior area is a black mass with spots of white. This represents superinfection with otomycosis. To the far left inferiorly is yellow-green mucopus covering the exposed mucosa of the tympanic cavity. In the inferior center portion of the photograph is a reddish-pink area of inflamed mucosa. To the right and inferior to this red mass is a relatively dry, white-tan colored structure, which is the remnant of the posterior-bony external auditory canal under which is probably the facial nerve. Initial treatment is to physically clean the cavity and then to instruct the patient to irrigate the cavity profusely with large amounts (1 cupful) of body-temperature vinegar four times daily. After a few days, when the cavity is free of discharge, treatment with an ear drop or powder containing a steroid and antibiotic is used to reduce inflammation and polypoid changes. Definitive treatment involves revision of the tympanoplasty, mastoidectomy, and reconstruction of the posterior bony external auditory canal as described by Pulec and Reams.[1]

Reference

1. Pulec JL, Reims CL. Reconstruction of radical mastoid cavities: methods and results. *Otolaryngol Clin North Am.* 1977;10(3):529–540.

134

Radical Mastoidectomy Cavity With Debris and Exposed Middle-Ear Mucosa

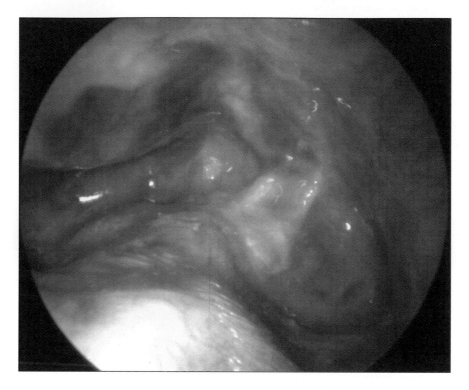

Fig 134–1

The otoscopic view is that of a left ear that has had a radical mastoidectomy. Infected epithelial debris covers the mastoid cavity and middle ear mucosa. At the bottom of the photograph is a skin-covered mound that is the remnant of the posterior external auditory canal bone. To the left is the mastoid cavity lined with dead, greenish, infected skin. In the center of the picture is the exposed epitympanic mucosa. To the right is the exposed mucous membrane of the tympanum and tubotympanum. The bacteria that usually produce the otorrhea are *staphylococcus aureus*, *pseudomonas*, and *proteus*. Treatment to eliminate the superficial infection is profuse frequent irrigation with body temperature vinegar. Revision tympanoplasty, mastoidectomy, and mastoid obliteration, usually with bone paste, can offer definitive relief.

135

Radical Mastoidectomy Cavity With Inflamed, Exposed Mucous Membrane

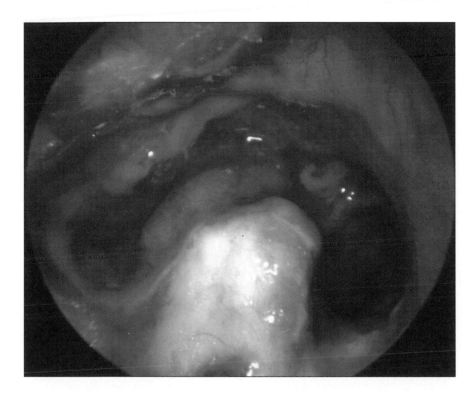

Fig 135–1

Patients with radical mastoidectomy cavities are still frequently seen despite the availability of intact posterior bony canal wall surgery. The otoscopic view is of the right ear of a patient who has had a radical mastoidectomy. The mucous membrane of the middle ear, epitympanum, and mastoid antrum are exposed and not covered with a graft. The mucous membrane is inflamed and covered with a mucoid discharge. At the center inferior portion of the picture, a remnant of the posterior external auditory canal lateral to the facial recess and facial nerve (which appears white from scarring) has epithelial debris on it as well as polypoid changes. Immediately to the right and superior is the cut end of the tensor tympani muscle and the cochleariform process. To the right of these structures is the inflamed mucous membrane of the tympanum and the tubotympanum. To the left and superior to the yellow-white mass is the exposed mucous membrane covering the medial wall of the antrum and mastoid. Although regular, intensive topical treatment with an ear drop or powder containing a steroid and antibiotic will control profuse otorrhea and odor, chronic discharge will continue until the mucous membrane has been covered. Definitive treatment involves revision of the tympanoplasty, mastoidectomy, and reconstruction of the posterior bony external auditory canal as described by Pulec and Reims.[1]

Reference

1. Pulec J, Reims CL. Reconstruction of radical mastoid cavities: methods and results. *Otolaryngol Clin North Am.* 1977;10(3):529–540.

SECTION X

Neoplasms

136

Benign Nevus of the External Auditory Canal

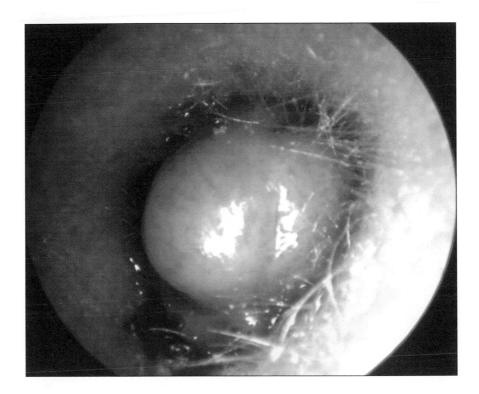

Fig 136–1

The otoscopic view is that of a left ear of a 61-year-old woman. A pink spherical mass fills the outer third of the external auditory canal. It was discovered serendipitously at the time of examination of chronic otitis media in the opposite ear. The mass in the left ear was completely asymptomatic. There was no otorrhea, pain, or hearing loss. The mass is covered with squamous epithelium and an air space can be seen posterior, superior, and inferior to the mass. Soft brown cerumen lines the external auditory canal. This neoplasm was removed using local anesthesia by excising the attachment from the anterior external auditory canal wall. The lesion was totally removed and found to be a benign nevus. The skin in the base was cauterized to con-

trol bleeding. The remaining portion of the external auditory canal skin was normal and the tympanic membrane was intact and completely normal. The canal and surgical site completely healed within 1 month. Differential diagnosis includes inflammatory polyp, encephalocele, foreign body granuloma, and a variety of benign and malignant neoplasms. Osteoma or exostoses usually have the appearance of paler skin covering hard bone. An inflammatory polyp would more commonly have a history of otorrhea and hearing loss. Adenoid-cystic carcinoma of the ceruminous glands characteristically is painful and exquisitely tender to the touch. Preoperative imaging is desirable and histopathologic examination is required in every case.

137

Facial Nerve Neuroma

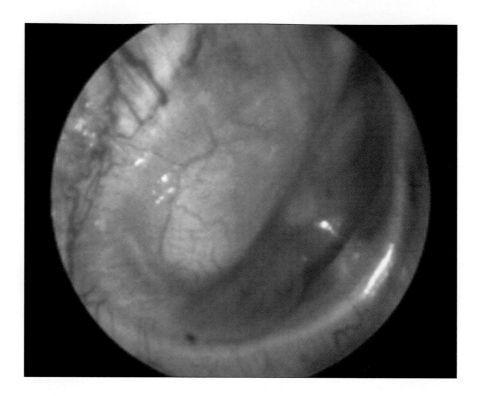

Fig 137–1

Facial nerve neuroma is an uncommon tumor that occurs with equal frequency in all segments of the facial nerve from the brain stem to the face. Tumors that originate in the tympanic portion of the nerve expand into the tympanum and produce symptoms of fullness of the ear and conductive hearing loss. The otoscopic appearance demonstrated in this right ear is typical of facial nerve neuroma. The pale, meaty, encapsulated globular tumor expands from the facial nerve and touches the posterior-superior quadrant of the tympanic membrane on its medial side. This otoscopic view reveals an intact tympanic membrane with bulging of the posterior-superior portion from pressure of the yellow-pink capsule of the tumor. The malleus can be seen from the umbo at the center of the drum head to the short process near the superior edge. An area of tympanum filled

with air can be seen inferior to the tumor in the posterior-inferior quadrant. A slightly more reddish lobe of the tumor extends anterior to the main mass immediately inferior to the umbo, and an air-containing space can be seen in the anterior-inferior quadrant. In this case a lobe of the tumor causes the tympanic membrane in the anterior-superior quadrant to bulge. This tumor's position in the posterior-superior part of the ear, as well as its pale appearance, helps differentiate it from a glomus tumor, which has a deep bluish red color and is seen more commonly arising from the hypotympanum. Diagnosis is confirmed by thin-section computed tomography and magnetic resonance imaging with gadolinium enhancement. The transcanal approach is to be avoided during surgical removal so that the tympanic membrane is maintained intact without adhesion or scar.

138

Mixed Adenoma of the Middle Ear*

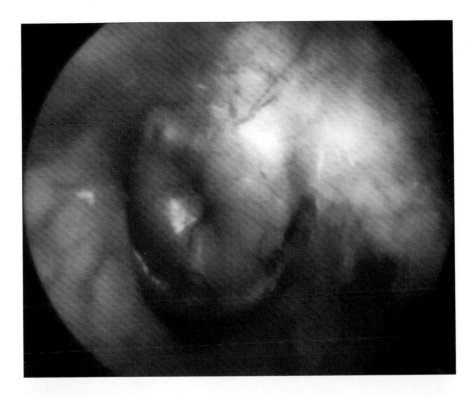

Fig 138–1

This picture shows a mixed adenoma of the left middle ear. The patient had decreased hearing, tinnitus, and fullness in the ear. Otoscopy revealed an opaque, pale, diffusely bulging tympanic membrane with increased vascularity. Anatomic structures remained well defined. The drum seems to be displaced laterally by a mass within the tympanum. Pneumatic otoscopy showed no mobility of the drum and computed tomography (CT) showed a nonvascular soft tissue mass confined to the middle ear. A tumor was suspected.

Surgical treatment included a complete mastoidectomy and extended facial recess approach. The bony external auditory canal was removed with a drill and the membranous external canal and the posterior aspect of the tympanic membrane were reflected anteriorly for optimal exposure. The tumor was attached to the promontory and filled the entire middle ear, but was easily peeled from the bony structures. The posterior canal wall was rebuilt using hydroxylapatite. The patient has remained recurrence free with normal hearing for the past 7 years. The last otoscopic examination was unremarkable.

Adenomatous tumors of the middle ear and mastoid can be classified as mixed or papillary tumors. Mixed-type tumors, such as the one in the picture, remain confined to the middle ear and mastoid, showing a propensity for extensive local damage and a tendency to recur. Therapy should include surgical excision and long-term follow-up.

Papillary type tumors are aggressive. They can cause temporal bone destruction and commonly show facial nerve involvement. Intracranial invasion is not uncommon and carries a poorer prognosis. Surgical intervention is recommended, but when impossible, radiation treatment is suggested.

*Chapter contributed by Ford Albritton, BS, and Armando Lenis, MD, Section of Otology, Scott & White Clinic, Texas A&M University Health Sciences Center, Temple, Texas.

Cavernous Hemangioma of the Tympanic Membrane*

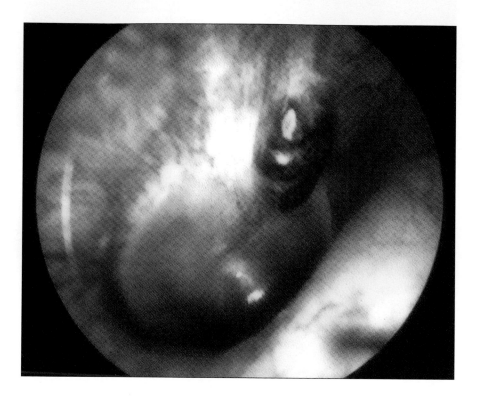

Fig 139–1

This photograph demonstrates a surgeon's view of a cavernous hemangioma of the left eardrum. The lesion was found serendipitously during a routine physical examination and known to be present and unchanged for over 10 years. At the time of examination the patient was completely asymptomatic with normal audiologic findings. The lesion is easily recognized by its color and its smooth, soft, well-defined multi-nodular appearance. These are rare tumors. A review of the literature over the last 20 years uncovered only three described cases. The most accepted treatment involved excision of the lesion with subsequent tympanoplasty. Other modalities of treatment suggested include photocoagulation with the yttrium-aluminum-garnet (YAG) laser and steroid injection.

*Chapter contributed by Ford Albritton, BS, and Armando Lenis, MD, Section of Otology, Scott & White Clinic, Texas A&M University Health Sciences Center, Temple, Texas.

140

Attic Angioma

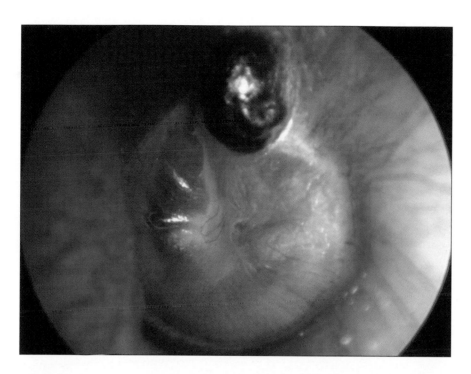

Fig 140–1

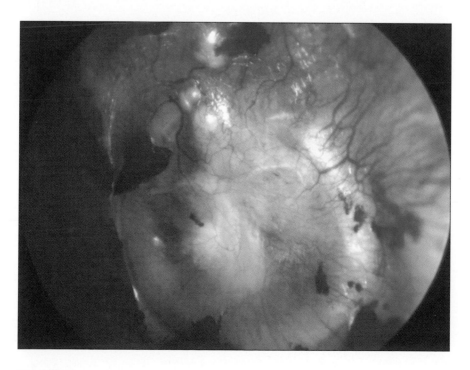

Fig 140–2

The upper photograph is an otoscopic view of the left ear of a 47-year-old man with no complaints and normal hearing. The blue globular mass protruding from the posterior part of Shrapnel's membrane was discovered on a routine otoscopic examination. The lesion was surgically removed and the resulting perforation was grafted with temporalis fascia. The photograph below demonstrates the otoscopic view of the same ear 6 years after surgery. Healing is excellent and hearing remained normal.

The differential diagnosis includes traumatic hematoma, hemangioma, cholesterol granulatoma, glomus tumor, or foreign body granuloma. Less likely possibilities based on the dark blue coloration might be meningioma or acoustic neuroma. Preoperative imaging with thin-section computerized tomography and magnetic resonance imaging with and without gadolinium enhancement will define the extent of the tumor. In this case, transcanal enucleation of a small neoplasm was possible.

141

Glomus Tumor of the Left Ear*

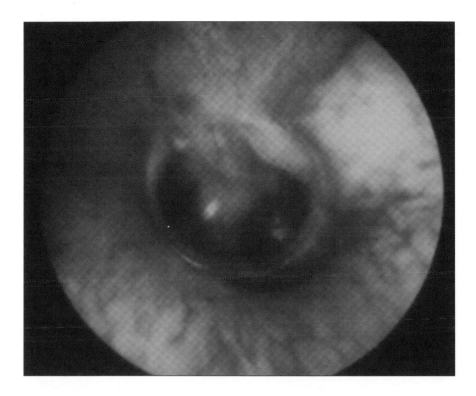

Fig 141–1

The otoscopic photograph is of the left ear and it shows a glomus tumor. The patient complained of progressively worsening throbbing with occasional pulsatile ringing in the left ear for 6 months. On physical examination she was found to have an abnormal eardrum with the classic sign of the "rising sun" behind the eardrum. A glomus tympanicum tumor, a glomus tumor limited to the middle ear, was found to be present when the tumor was studied with digital subtraction angiography. The blood supply was from the terminal branch of the ascending pharyngeal artery branch of the external carotid artery on the left side. Computed tomography (CT) with high definition and magnification indicated that there was no destruction of the mastoid bone and there was only partial filling of the hypotympanum. Without good imaging of the interior of the jugular bulb and vein there is no way to differentiate a tympanicum from a jugular glomus tumor.

The limited tumor allowed a transcanal removal after removal of the lateral wall of the hypotympanum. The blood supply to the tumor was controlled with the bipolar cautery. The tumor was removed in one piece. The eardrum was replaced in its proper anatomic position.

In the assessment of glomus tumors it is helpful to investigate the size of the tumor by means of digital subtraction angiography as well as by CT of the temporal bones. Surgery is favored in most cases, but some large glomulus tumors may be treated with radiotherapy in centers where it is felt that arresting tumor growth is a reasonable alternative to the risk of morbidity that may occur with total removal.

*This chapter was contributed by Tibor Ruff, MD, Division of Otolaryngology Head and Neck Surgry, Scott & White Clinic, Texas A&M University Health Sciences Center, Temple, Texas.

142
Glomus Jugulare Tumor

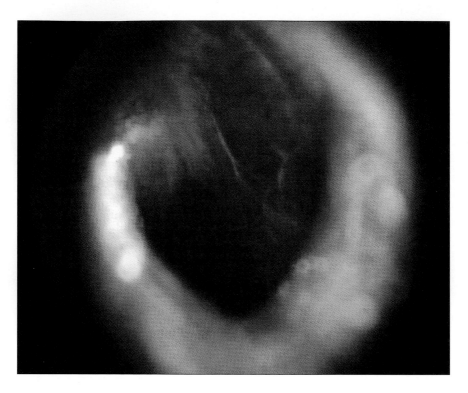

Fig 142–1

Unless an area of promontory that appears normal can be seen completely around the tumor, it is impossible to otoscopically differentiate a glomus jugulare from a glomus tympanicum tumor. In the otoscopic view of this right tympanic membrane, an obvious cranberry-red mass can be seen through the tympanic membrane in the posterior-inferior quadrant of the tympanum. The tumor extends from under the annulus and its full extent cannot be determined by otoscopy. The anterior half of the pars tensa has increased vascularity as well as lines from old scars. A small, darkened area superior to the red mass represents the round-window niche. To the trained otologist, this view establishes a diagnosis of glomus tumor. Use of a pneumatic otoscope can elicit Brown's sign, first described by Lester Brown. Examinations include audiometric and vestibular tests to establish involvement of function, thin-

section computerized tomography to determine bone destruction and extent of the lesion, and magnetic resonance imaging (MRI) with gadolinium and MRA to determine the size of the tumor and whether it is a tympanicum or glomus tumor. A retrograde jugular venogram is usually necessary to precisely demonstrate the position of the tumor within the jugular vein. A transcanal approach is indicated only for the smallest isolated tumor in the center of the promontory, and transcanal biopsy is never indicated because it will lead to an adhesion of the tympanic membrane to the tumor and hamper the opportunity to obtain normal hearing. Complete tumor removal through the extended facial recess and retrofacial recess approaches through the mastoid allows preservation of the external auditory canal. Blood transfusion is rarely necessary and extradural tumors are removed with outpatient surgery.

143

Squamous Carcinoma of the External Auditory Canal

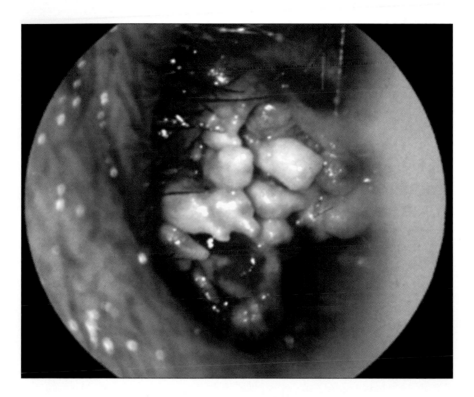

Fig 143–1

Although the majority of tumors that originate within the external auditory canal are benign inflammatory polyps related to ear infections, a variety of benign and malignant tumors occurs in the ear canal. The photograph is of a right ear, showing the external auditory canal containing squamous cell carcinoma. The mass appears to be attached to the anterior canal wall skin. Hair is seen extending from the posterior-superior ear canal skin. The surface of the tumor has white irregular protuberances and an appearance that suggests carcinoma. At the inferior portion of the mass there is evidence of a recent biopsy. Carcinoma of the external auditory canal is frequently accompanied by persistent otalgia. Unusually severe persistent pain and tenderness are characteristic of adenoid cystic carcinoma. Diagnosis should be made without delay and treatment involves wide surgical excision of the external auditory canal, tympanic membrane, condyle of the mandible, and total parotidectomy (canalectomy) as described by Pulec.[1] In some cases, temporal bone resection and radical neck dissection may be required.

Reference

1. Pulec, JL. Glandular tumors of the external auditory canal. *Laryngoscope.* 1977;87(10):1601–1612.

144

Fibrous Dysplasia of the Temporal Bone

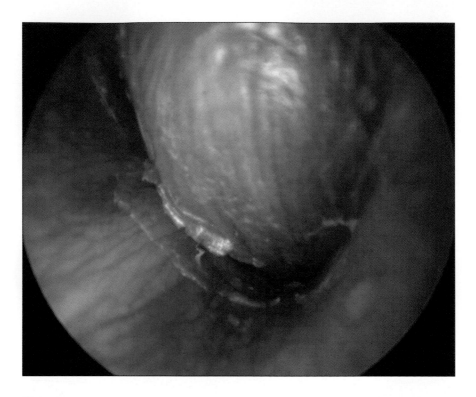

Fig 144–1

The otoscopic view is that of a left ear canal in a 24-year-old man. A hard, slow-growing, bonelike mass is seen extending from the superior external auditory canal wall. Only a small slit of the external canal opening remains at the inferior edge of the canal. Treatment involves the repeated conservative surgical excision of the obstructing fibrous dysplasia and of abnormal bone within the external auditory canal and, in some cases, also in the middle ear. Repeated surgery is required as needed every few months or years, depending on the rate of growth.

145

Osteoma of the External Auditory Canal

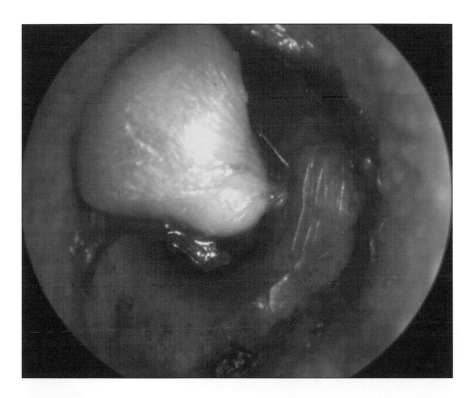

Fig 145–1

Osteomas are benign neoplasms that may extend beyond the immediate region such as into the mastoid.[1] Imaging with computerized tomography usually reveals the nature of the lesion. The solitary tumor seen in this otoscopic view of a left ear extends from the anterior canal wall. It is connected by a relatively thin neck of bone that can be fractured by pressure from a curet or Rosen elevator in the office. The skin of the canal will promptly heal over the bone at the fracture site.

Reference

1. Schuknecht HF. *Pathology of the ear.* Cambridge, Mass: Harvard University Press; 1974:383.

146

Large Osteoma of the External Auditory Canal

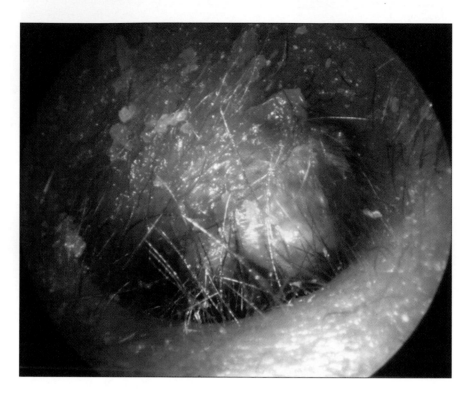

Fig 146–1

The otoscopic view is that of a right ear of a 40-year-old man. He complained of obstruction and hearing loss. The bone-hard mass fills the ear canal and is mobile on palpation. The diagnosis of osteoma was confirmed by computerized tomography. The tumor was removed easily by cutting the skin around the fractured neck at its attachment to the anterior bony canal wall. The skin quickly healed over the bone after the osteoma was removed.

SECTION XI

Congenital Anomalies

147

Congenital Atresia of the External Auditory Canal

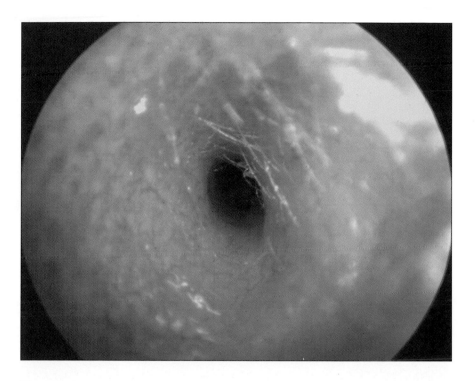

Fig 147–1

The otoscopic view is that of stenosis of the external auditory canal on the left. The opening is one tenth the normal size and ends in a blunted skin-covered, bony obstruction 5 mm from the lateral surface. There is no tympanic membrane and the bony external auditory canal is absent. Anomalies of this type can be unilateral or bilateral. They can be associated with microtia of varying degrees or the pinna can otherwise be completely normal. Three factors must be considered by the otologist in each case[1]: (1) The presence of a portion of the external auditory canal lined with squamous epithelium medial to the obstructed external auditory canal must be excluded; should such a pouch be present, it is identified by thin-section computerized tomography (CT) and timely corrective surgery is mandatory. (2) Hearing must be provided promptly by surgery or amplification, so that the individual can learn speech and become educated. (3) The

cosmetic appearance should be improved with the creation of a pinna by plastic surgery or use of a bone-anchored prosthesis. Construction of an auditory canal and tympanoplasty requires special skill. This surgery is usually performed by only a few otologic surgeons who have a large experience and special interest in congenital ear anomalies. Reconstruction of the ear canal and hearing is recommended for both bilateral and unilateral cases. Reasonable success for the attainment of near-normal hearing can be expected. Patients and their families are usually given the choice of having an auricle created by plastic surgical techniques using rib cartilage or an appliance anchored to the side of the skull to which a prosthetic ear is attached.

Reference

1. Pulec JL, Freedman HM. Management of congenital ear anomalies. *Laryngoscope*. 1978;88(3):420–434.

148

Congenital Malformation: Abnormal Position of the Malleus

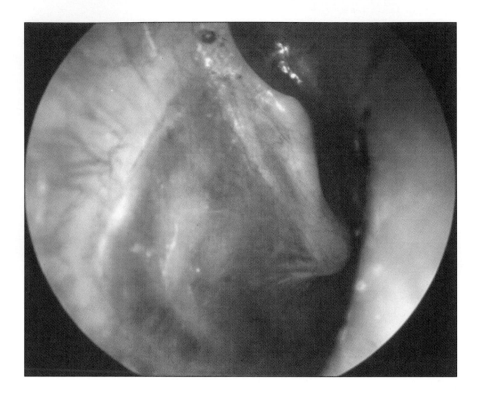

Fig 148–1

The otoscopic view is that of a right ear with malformation and malposition of the malleus. The external auditory canal is normal and the pars tensa is intact. The malleus is malformed with a shortened lateral process and elongated neck. The umbo and inferior portion of the manubrium are malposi-tioned more anteriorly than normal. The ear may or may not have a hearing loss. If a conductive hearing loss is present, tympanoplasty performed under a local anesthetic may be desirable. Use of a hearing aid is an alternative method of treatment.

149

Congenital Anomaly: Middle-Ear Malformation

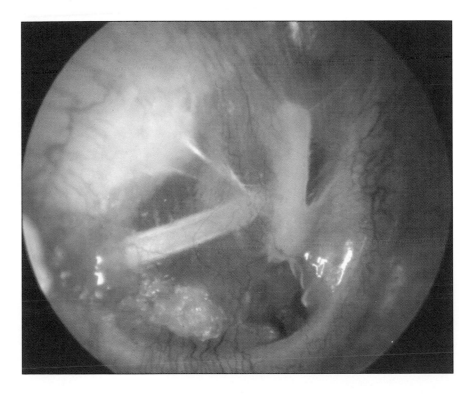

Fig 149–1

The otoscopic view is that of the right ear of a patient with conductive hearing loss bilaterally. The tympanic membrane is intact but shows evidence of previous infection and healing with a two-layered membrane. A triangular-shaped part of normal-appearing pars tensa extends from the umbo to the anterior annulus. The obvious abnormality is the shortened and thickened vertically placed manubrium of the malleus and the inferiorly placed chorda tympani nerve. The chorda tympani nerve is seen through the tympanic membrane crossing the tympanum at the largest diameter of the tympanic ring. A small mass of golden-colored cerumen overlies the exit of the chorda tympani nerve from the posterior canniculus. The caliber of the nerve is larger than normal. Treatment is tympanoplasty with ossicular reconstruction.

150

Congenital Malformation of the Middle Ear

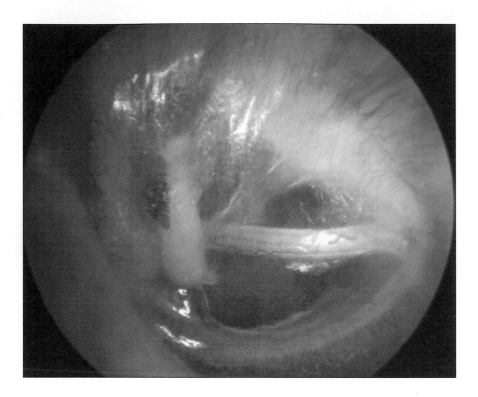

Fig 150–1

The otoscopic view is that of the left ear of the same patient as shown in the previous chapter. The appearance is similar to that of the right ear. Surgical correction by tympanoplasty can often eliminate the conductive hearing loss. Any part of the ossicu-lar chain can be involved with fixation or abnormality. Great care must be taken to avoid injury to the facial nerve, which often has an anomalous course and position in the tympanum.

Index

B

Bacilli, acid-fast stain, 135
Barotrauma, 47
Blue eardrum, 62, 63, 64, 121, 151
"Blue ear," hemotympanum, 62, 63
Brain abscess, 83, 118, 120
Bronchitis, chronic, 31
Brown, Lester, 184

C

Canalectomy, 185
Candida, 27
Carcinoma
    adenoid-cystic, 177
    external auditory canal, 185
Cerumen
    impacted, 19
    removal, 19
Cerumenex, 19
Cholesteatoma, 85, 86, 101
    attic, 78, 86
        atelectasis, 125
        and blue eardrum, 121–122
        chronic suppurative otitis media, 83, 84, 85, 92, 117,
            118–119, 120, 121–122
        in epitympanum, anterior, 127–128
        erosion, superior bony canal wall, 124
        facial palsy, 120
        and polyp, 121–122
        recurrence prevention, 123, 124, 126, 127–128
        and tympanosclerosis, 118–119, 120, 123, 126
    auditory canal, external, 31
    chronic suppurative otitis media, 83, 84, 85, 94
    congenital middle ear, 101
    pearls, 168
    recurrence prevention, 117, 123, 124, 126, 127–128
    and tympanosclerosis, 118–119, 120, 123, 126, 133
    tympanum, extension into, 129
Chorda tympani, 3, 5
Chronic otitis media. *See under* Otitis
Ciprofloxacin, 22
Circulatory system, 3, 4
Cleft palate
    and perforation, 77
    serous otitis media, 69, 74
Cochlea, fenestrae cochleae, fossula, 5
Cochlear window. *See* Fenestrae cochleae
Cold, common, 39, 47
Conductive hearing loss. *See under* Hearing loss
Congenital anomalies
    atresia, external auditory canal, 191
    malleus malposition, 192
    middle ear malformation, 193–194
Corticosteroids, 49
Cow's milk products, 76
Cresylate, 25
Cysts, following myringoplasty, 167

D

Decongestants, 39, 40, 42, 61

Diabetes mellitus, 23
DiBartolomeo, Joseph R., 168
Dysplasia, temporal bone, 186

E

Ear drops, 62, 63, 115, 121, 150, 171, 173
"Eardrum, blue," 62
Ecchymosis, 47
Edema, auditory canal, external, 29
Encephalocele, 83, 177
Epithelitis, tympanic membrane graft, 49
Eustachian tube catheter, serous otitis media, 57
Eustachian tube obstruction, serous otitis media, 57
Exostoses, 32, 177
    distinguished from osteomas, 33
    hearing loss, 36
    infection, 36
    nonobstructing, 33, 34
    obstructing, 35, 36
    surgery, 33, 35, 36

F

Fenestrae cochleae fossula, 5
Fever, 22
Fistulae, labyrinthine, 84, 85, 92, 118, 120
Fracture. *See also* Trauma
    crura, 160
    temporal bone
        with conductive hearing loss, 156, 157
        with crura fracture, 160
        with displacement, 152
        healed, 152, 153, 154, 155, 157, 158
        with hemorrhage, 154
        with incus dislocation, 161, 163
        posttympanoplasty, 162
        with tympanic membrane perforation, 154–155,
            163–164
Furunculosis, 22–23
    and diabetes mellitus, 23

G

Gamma globulin medication, 62, 63
Glomus tumor, 178, 182, 183
    jugulare, 183
"Glue ear," 60
Grafts. *See* Surgery
Granuloma
    cholesterol, 151, 182
        and blue eardrum, 121
        serous otitis media, 57, 62, 63, 64
    foreign body, 177, 182

H

Hearing, second-stage reconstruction, 85, 114, 116, 117,
        119, 121, 123, 124, 125, 126, 127, 129, 132, 133
Hearing aids, 191, 192
Hearing loss
    amplification, 191, 192

tuberculosis, 134–135
  and tympanosclerosis, 83, 84, 85, 90, 96, 111
  Type I, 83, 89
  tympanosclerosis, 105
effects of, 110
and labyrinthitis, viral, 39
myringitis, bullous, 39
progressive, 115
purulent stage, 43
secretory, 60
serous, 39, 47, 57–78
  atelectasis, 53, 54
  cholesterol granuloma, 57, 62, 63, 64
  with cleft palate, 69, 74
  hemotympanum, 151
  mechanisms leading to, 57
  and neomembrane, healed, 61
  and pars tensa retraction, 59
  recurrent, 111
  and tympanosclerosis, 61, 65
  Valsalva maneuver, 57, 61
suppurative, 79–122. *See also* acute, suppurative in
    this section
viral, 39, 60
Otomycosis
  acetic irrigation, 25, 26
  flourishing, 27–28
  and mastoidectomy, radical, 171
  with pus, 25
Otorrhea, 29, 44, 50, 76, 83, 145, 173
  bacteria, 172
  cerebrospinal, 83
  mucous, 63
  purulent, 134
Otosclerosis
  chronic suppurative otitis media, 90
  clinical confirmation, 103
  footplate, 103

P

Paget disease, 90
Pain. *See* Otalgia
Palsy, facial, 120
Papillary-type tumors, 179
Paralysis, facial, 85, 92, 118, 163
Parotidectomy, 185
Pars flaccida, 4
Pars tensa. *See* Tympanic membrane
Pathology, atelectasis, 51–52
Pearl, epithelial, 167
Pediatrics
  bathing, 76
  cholesteatoma, 102
  foreign body, auditory canal, external, 21
  fracture, temporal bone, healed, 158
  "glue ear," 60
  myringostomy
    granulation tissue formation, 75
    grommet ventilation, 66
    swimming/bathing, 76

otitis media
  acute suppurative, 40
  secretory, 60
  "string of pearls," 168
  swimming, 76
  tuberculous chronic otitis media, 134–135
Penicillin, beta-lactamase-resistant, 22
Penicillium, 27
Perforation
  after grommet insertion, 77
  blast injury, 149
  cholesteatoma, 84, 85, 131–132
    attic, 84, 85
  concussion trauma, 145
  dry central tympanic membrane, 95, 98–99, 100
    with squamous epithelium in tympanum, 113–114
    tympanosclerosis, 100, 104
  hair microperforation, 96
  healed, with neomembrane retracted, 108–109
  with hemorrhage, 154
  ossicular fixation, 107
  otosclerosis, footplate, 103
  pars tensa, 131–132
  Pulec-Deguine Type I chronic suppurative otitis
      media, 83, 84, 89
  Pulec-Deguine Type III chronic suppurative otitis
      media, 83, 84, 91, 111–112, 131
  Pulec-Deguine Type IV chronic suppurative otitis
      media, 84, 85
  Pulec-Deguine Type V chronic suppurative otitis
      media, 93
  Pulec-Deguine Type VI chronic suppurative otitis
      media, 133
  slag burn, 97
  spontaneous healing, 145, 146, 148, 150, 154
  with squamous epithelium in tympanum, 113–114,
      115, 116
  trauma
    concussion, 145–146
    fracture, temporal bone, 154, 155, 163–164
    with hemorrhage, 154
    Q-tip injury, 147
    temporal bone fracture, 154, 155, 163–164
  tympanosclerosis
    dry central tympanic membrane, 100, 104, 113
    malleus fixed, 106
    ossicular fixation, 107
Per-Lee, John, 69
Phenylpropanolamine, 39, 40, 42, 47, 61
Pinna microtia, 191
Plastic surgery, 191
Pneumococci, 39
Pneumococcus, 41, 42
Polyps, 177
  and attic cholesteatoma, 121
  and blue eardrum, 121
  granulation tissue, 84, 85
  Pulec-Deguine Type V chronic suppurative otitis
      media, 130
Promontory, tympanic, 5
Prostheses, 114
  ear, 191

Prostheses (*continued*)
partial ossicular replacement prosthesis (PORP), 161, 163
total ossicular replacement prosthesis (TORP), 161
tympanoplasty, 105, 109, 111
Wright eustachian tube, 111
Wehr's hydroxyapatite, 152, 155, 162
Wright eustachian tube, 111
Proteus, 171
Protympanum, 5. *See also* Tubotympanum
Pseudomonas, 171
Pure-tone audiometry, concussion perforation, 145

Q

Q-tip injury, 147
Quinolone, 22

R

Radiation treatment, 179, 183
Reconstruction, external auditory canal, 191
Rivinus notch, 4

S

Salpingitis, viral, 42
Serous otitis media. *See under* Otitis
Short process of malleus. *See* lateral process under Malleus
Sinusitis, chronic, 77
Stapedectomy, 83, 90, 103
Stapes, 3
Staphylococcus aureus, 22, 23, 172
Steroids, 27, 29, 30, 48, 76, 83, 121, 130, 150, 171, 173, 180
Streptococci, 39, 42
beta-hemolytic, 40, 77
Stria membrana, 4
"Surfers ear," 33
Surgery
adenoidectomy, 76, 77
adhesion prevention, 91, 105, 113–114, 115, 116, 119, 132
attic cholesteatoma, 117, 170
Bondi modified radical mastoidectomy, 170
canalectomy, 185
cholesteatoma removal, 85, 86, 94, 101, 102
basement membrane, 89, 129
chronic suppurative otitis media management, 86
classification, 86
dry central perforation, 95, 99, 100, 104, 113–114
exostoses, 33, 35, 36
flap, tympanomeatal, 83, 90, 121, 129, 155
grafts
homograft tympanic membranes, 52, 70, 100, 110, 115, 169
lateralization, 169
myringoplasty, 95, 99
fascia graft, 169
tympanoplasty, 105
homograft, 104
homograft tympanic membranes, 52, 70, 100, 110, 115,

169
mastoid, blue eardrum, 62
mastoid drainage, 85
mastoidectomy, 65, 85, 113, 117, 132
Bondi modified radical, 170
extended facial recess approach, 179
and myringotomy, 78
radical, 85
with debris, 172
with inflammation, 173
modified, 170
with mucous membrane exposed, 173
with otomycosis, 171
surgical management system, 86
transcanal, 124
tympanoplasty, 125
and tympanoplasty, 121–122, 129, 130, 133, 134, 171, 172, 173
and tympanoplasty and myringoplasty, 123, 126, 127–128
tympanosclerosis, 170
and type IV myringoplasty, 118–119
and type IV tympanoplasty, 120
for myringitis, 48
myringoplasty, 49, 52, 54, 71, 77, 85, 97, 103, 154
concussion perforation, 145
cysts, 167
epithelial pearl, 167
fascia graft, 169
graft, 95
transcanal, 104
and tympanoplasty, 123
and tympanoplasty and mastoidectomy, 123, 126, 127–128
tympanosclerosis, 167
type III, and tympanoplasty, 111–112, 131
type IV, and tympanoplasty and mastoidectomy, 118–119
myringostapedopexy, 109
myringostapedopexy creation, 9
ossiculoplasty, 163
parotidectomy, 185
plastic surgery, 191
postauricular incision, 132
preoperative
appraisal, 86
myringotomy, 111
prosthesis, 114
partial ossicular replacement prosthesis (PORP), 161, 163
total ossicular replacement prosthesis (TORP), 161
tympanoplasty, 105, 109
Wright eustachian tube, 111
Wehr's hydroxyapatite, 152, 155, 162
Pulec type III, 131
Pulec type V, 130
Pulec type VI, 123, 133
reconstruction, 121
ossicular, 9, 83, 90, 116, 120, 123, 124, 125, 126, 127–128, 129, 133, 152, 158, 160, 162
posterior bony external auditory canal, 171, 173
repeat, 186

Roman numeral classification, 86
Silastic adhesion prevention, 91, 105, 113–114, 115, 116, 119, 132
slag burn, 97
stapedectomy, 83, 90, 103
tonsillectomy, 76, 77
transcanal, 178, 182, 184
  mastoidectomy, 124
  myringoplasty, 104
  tympanoplasty, 104, 115, 125, 156
tympanoplasty, 14, 26, 35, 85, 86, 87–88, 137, 139, 141, 154, 155, 157, 158, 159, 162
  attic cholesteatoma, 117
  chronic suppurative otitis media, 85, 86, 87–88
  congenital atresia, external auditory canal, 191
  hemangioma of tympanic membrane, cavernous, 180
  malleus malposition, congenital, 192
  and mastoidectomy, 121–122, 125, 129, 130, 133, 134, 171, 172, 173
  with mastoidectomy, 117
  middle ear malformation, 193–194
  and myringoplasty and mastoidectomy, 123, 126, 127–128
  and myringotomy, 78
  one-stage, 106
  ossicle placement, 107
  prosthesis, 105, 109
    Wright eustachian tube, 111
  by reconstruction, 109
  revision, 172
  squamous epithelium in tympanum, 116
  surgical management system, 85, 86
  transcanal, 104, 115, 125, 156
  two-stage, 105, 107, 116, 119
  tympanosclerosis, 105, 116
  type I, 163
    (after Wulstein), 89
  type IV, and mastoidectomy, 120
    and type IV myringoplasty, 118–119
  type VI, 123, 126, 127–128, 133
"Swimmer's ear," 29

T

Thrombosis, venous, 83
Tinnitus, 147
  adenoma of middle ear, mixed, 179
  concussion perforation, 145
  keratinized epithelial folds, 24
  labyrinthitis, 39
  otomycosis, 27
Tonsillectomy, 76, 77
Tonsils, serous otitis media, 59
Trauma
  barotrauma, 47
  dislocation, incus, 161, 163
  dry central tympanic membrane perforation, 95
  fracture
    crura, 160
    temporal bone
      with conductive hearing loss, 156, 157

  with crura fracture, 160
  with displacement, 152
  healed, 152, 153, 154, 155, 157
  with hemorrhage, 154
  with incus dislocation, 161, 163
  old, 153
  posttympanoplasty, 162
  with stapes capitulum dislocation, 160
  with tympanic membrane perforation, 154–155, 163–164
hemotympanum, 151
perforation
  blast injury, 149
  concussion, 145–146
  Q-tip injury, 147
  spontaneous healing, 145–146, 148, 150, 154
Travel, air. *See* Air travel
Trichloracetic acid, 50
Tuberculosis, 134–135
  hemotympanum, 151
Tubotympanum, 3, 5. *See also* Protympanum
Tympani anticus, 4
Tympanic membrane
  normal, 3
  pars tensa, 4
  pathology
    aerotitis, 47
    atelectasis, 51–52
    barotrauma, 47
    epithelitis, of graft, 49
    myringitis, 48, 50
  umbo, 4
Tympanic spine, 4
Tympani posticus, 4
Tympanomeatal flap surgery, 83, 90, 121, 129, 155
Tympanoplasty, 14, 26, 35, 85, 86, 87–88, 137, 139, 141, 154, 155, 157, 158, 159, 162
  basement membrane, 107, 129
  chronic suppurative otitis media, 85, 86, 87–88
  congenital atresia, external auditory canal, 191
  graft, 105
    homograft, 104
  homograft, 104
  malleus malposition, congenital, 192
  and mastoidectomy, 121–122, 125, 129, 130, 133, 134, 171, 172, 173
  with mastoidectomy, 117
  middle ear malformation, 193–194
  and myringoplasty and mastoidectomy, 123, 126, 127–128
  and myringotomy, 78
  one-stage, 106
  ossicle placement, 107
  prosthesis, 105, 109
    Wright eustachian tube, 111
  Pulec type IV, 64, 65, 121–122
  by reconstruction, 109
  revision, 172
  squamous epithelium in tympanum, 116
  surgical management system, 85, 86
  transcanal, 104, 115, 125, 156
  two-stage, 105, 107, 116, 119
  tympanosclerosis, 105, 116